YOUR LAST NURSING CLASS: HOW TO LAND YOUR FIRST NURSING JOB

YOUR LAST NURSING CLASS: HOW TO LAND YOUR FIRST NURSING JOB

The ultimate guide to landing your first nursing job...and your next !

Beth Hawkes MSN, RN-BC

ISBN-13: 9780692829318
ISBN-10: 0692829318
Library of Congress Control Number: 2017904427
Your Last Nursing Class, Bakersfield, CA

10.99

*With love and gratitude to my husband,
Bob with his unfailing patience.*

Contents

Preface · xiii
What This Book Will Do for You · · · · · · · · · xiv

1 Job Outlook · **1**
Job Market for New Grads · · · · · · · · · · · · · 1
Nursing Shortage? · · · · · · · · · · · · · · · · · · 2
Nursing Shortage Redefined · · · · · · · · · · · · 3
Skill Acquisition · · · · · · · · · · · · · · · · · · · 6

2 Application Process · · · · · · · · · · · · · · · · **9**
Follow the Process · · · · · · · · · · · · · · · · · · 10
Don't Wait to Apply—You'll Be Late! · · · · · · 11
Required versus Preferred · · · · · · · · · · · · · 13
Common Errors · · · · · · · · · · · · · · · · · · · 14
References and Letters of
Recommendations · · · · · · · · · · · · · · · · · · 15
Prehire Application Tests · · · · · · · · · · · · · 17
Persevere · 18

3 Insider Tips and Strategies · · · · · · · · · · · **21**
Know the Players · · · · · · · · · · · · · · · · · · 21
Know What Counts · · · · · · · · · · · · · · · · · 23

Know What Nurse Managers Want · · · · · · · · 24
Know Your Potential Employer · · · · · · · · · · 26
Job Postings · 28
Elevator Speech· · · · · · · · · · · · · · · · · · · 31
Missed Opportunity · · · · · · · · · · · · · · · · 33
Practice, Practice · · · · · · · · · · · · · · · · · · 34
Get Connected, Stay Connected · · · · · · · · 36
4 It's Not All about You · · · · · · · · · · · · · · · 37
Change Your Point of View · · · · · · · · · · · · 37
Think Like a Boss · · · · · · · · · · · · · · · · · · 39
5 Networking · 43
What Is Networking Really?· · · · · · · · · · · · 44
Networking Myths· · · · · · · · · · · · · · · · · · 44
Leverage Your Network· · · · · · · · · · · · · · 46
Opportunity Strikes· · · · · · · · · · · · · · · · · 48
Employee Referrals · · · · · · · · · · · · · · · · 49
6 Certifications · 51
Certifications for New Grad Nurses · · · · · · 53
Basic Life Support (BLS) · · · · · · · · · · · · · 53
ECG Courses · 54
Advanced Cardiovascular Life-Support
Course (ACLS)· 55
National Institutes of Health Stroke Scale
(NIHSS) · 56
Trauma Nursing Core Course (TNCC)· · · · · · 56
Emergency Nursing Pediatric Course
(ENPC)· 57
Pediatric Advanced Life-Support Course
(PALS)· 57

Neonatal Resuscitation Program (NRP) · · · · · 58

STABLE Program · 59

Final Tips on Certifications for New Grad
Nurses · 59

7 Tips for Student Nurses · · · · · · · · · · · · · · · · 61

Mind-set of a Successful RN · · · · · · · · · · · · · 62

Start Now · 63

Know Who's Who · 63

Work as a Nursing Assistant or PCT · · · · · · · 64

Be a Superstar · 66

Write a Note to the Manager · · · · · · · · · · · · 66

Volunteer · 67

Network. Network. Network. · · · · · · · · · · · · 68

8 Standout Résumés · · · · · · · · · · · · · · · · · · · 71

Formatting Rules You Must Follow · · · · · · · · 73

Verbs and Tense · 76

Keywords · 76

Avoid Clichés · 77

Category Sequencing · · · · · · · · · · · · · · · · · · · 78

Customizing · 80

Optional: Objectives/Summary
Statements · 81

Qualifications, Certifications, and
Education · 82

You Have Skills · 83

What Are Hard Skills and Soft Skills? · · · · · · 83

Words Tell, Stories Sell · · · · · · · · · · · · · · · · · 84

Work History · 85

Volunteer · 85

Critique · 85
Checklist/Summary · · · · · · · · · · · · · · · 86
Creative Strategies · · · · · · · · · · · · · · · 86
Testimonials · 87

9 Cover Letters · · · · · · · · · · · · · · · · · · 91
Cover Letter Basics · · · · · · · · · · · · · · · 93
Opening · 96
Middle · 96
Closing · 97
Business Print Copy Format · · · · · · · · · · · 98
E-mail Format · 98
Wait to Hit Send · · · · · · · · · · · · · · · · · 99
Creative Strategies for Cover Letters · · · · · 100
Chapter Summary and Checklist · · · · · · · · 104

10 Essay Questions · · · · · · · · · · · · · · · · 107
How to Write a Nursing Application
Essay · 109
Follow Instructions · · · · · · · · · · · · · · · · 109
Allow Ample Time · · · · · · · · · · · · · · · · · 110
Be the Recruiter · · · · · · · · · · · · · · · · · · 110
Be a Good Fit · 112

11 Confidence: How to Have It · · · · · · · · 115
Wow Them with Confidence · · · · · · · · · · · 116
Step Onto Your Stage · · · · · · · · · · · · · · · 117
Confident Posture · · · · · · · · · · · · · · · · · 118
Strange Confidence-Building Exercise · · · · 118
Confident, Professional Appearance · · · · · · 119
Manage Your Nervousness · · · · · · · · · · · · 120
Confidence Specific to the Job
Requirements · 121

12 Interviews: General · · · · · · · · · · · · **123**

Be the Memorable One · · · · · · · · · · · · 124

Exude Confidence · · · · · · · · · · · · · · · 126

First Impressions · · · · · · · · · · · · · · · 128

What to Bring to Your Nursing Interview · · · 129

Portfolio · 130

If You Freeze During an Interview · · · · · · · 133

Preparation is the best prevention · · · · · · · 136

13 Video Interviews · · · · · · · · · · · · · · · **137**

Set the Stage for Your Video Interview · · · · 137

Lights, Camera, Action · · · · · · · · · · · · · 138

Dress for Success · · · · · · · · · · · · · · · · 139

Act the Part · · · · · · · · · · · · · · · · · · · 139

Technicalities · · · · · · · · · · · · · · · · · · 140

Not Live · 140

Prepare and Rehearse · · · · · · · · · · · · · 140

14 Behavioral Interview Questions · · · · · · · **141**

Prepare These Three Examples · · · · · · · · · 142

Rehearse · 144

Tell Us About Yourself · · · · · · · · · · · · · 145

Why Should We Hire You? · · · · · · · · · · · · 147

Why Should We Hire You?

Examples · 148

What's Your Best Strength? · · · · · · · · · · · 150

What are your best strengths?

Examples: · 151

Give an Example of a Time... · · · · · · · · · 152

Tell Us About a Conflict at Work · · · · · · · · 153

What's Your Greatest Weakness? · · · · · · · · 156

Your greatest weaknesses Examples · · · · · · 158

15 Situational Interview Questions · · · · · · · **161**

Principles of Situational Questions · · · · · · · 162

The Basic Clinical Scenario · · · · · · · · · · · · 163

Clinical Cues · 164

16 Closing the Interview and Beyond · · · · · **167**

What Questions Do You Have for Us? · · · · · 167

Bonus Question · 168

Things Never to Ask · · · · · · · · · · · · · · · · · 169

How to Stand Out · · · · · · · · · · · · · · · · · · · 169

Make Yourself Stand Out · · · · · · · · · · · · · · 171

The Waiting Game · · · · · · · · · · · · · · · · · · · 172

If You Don't Get the Job · · · · · · · · · · · · · · 172

17 Final Words and Bonus FAQs · · · · · · · · · **175**

Cold-Calling a Nurse Manager · · · · · · · · · · 176

After My Interview, When Should I Call
Back? · 178

I'm Older—What About Ageism? · · · · · · · · 180

Can I Ask for More Money as a New Grad? · · 184

What if I Have a DUI? · · · · · · · · · · · · · · · · · 187

What if I'm Offered Another Job While
Waiting to Hear Back? · · · · · · · · · · · · · · · · 190

Conclusion · 193

About the Author · 195

Suggested Readings · · · · · · · · · · · · · · · · · · 197

A warm welcome, my nursing friend! One thing is for sure: you are determined and goal oriented to have made it this far in nursing. Congratulations on your progress! Whether you are a nursing student, a new graduate, or an experienced nurse, I want to help you land that dream job.

This book is for the new graduate nurse who is ready to launch his or her nursing career and become the nurse he or she has always dreamed of becoming but first needs to land a job.

It's also for the experienced nurse who wants to change location or practice specialty but never learned how to write an effective résumé or cover letter or how to approach an interview. Those skills weren't particularly needed back in the day, but they are essential in today's competitive market.

You must learn how to:

- Compose a compelling cover letter (to make them want to read your résumé)
- Create a skills-based résumé that ensures you stand out (to get an interview)
- Conduct a memorable, impressive interview (to land the job)

Consider this book the last textbook of your final class, teaching you the skills you were not taught in nursing school. With over a decade's experience as a hiring manager, I will give you essential insider tips. What do nurse managers look for in a new hire? Did you know that there is an ideal new employee all nurse managers are looking for and want to hire? It does not necessarily have to do with experience. I will show you how to be that person in your résumé, cover letter, and interview.

Many examples are included throughout the book. Most are real-life conversations and testimonials I've had with nurses and students via e-mail and social media; others are compilations. All names have been changed.

WHAT THIS BOOK WILL DO FOR YOU

Landing a good job in a competitive environment takes key skills, proven strategies, and insider industry tips. Wherever you are in your career or job search, you will learn:

- Why your résumé is not about you—and why it's a mistake to think it is
- How to compose an elevator speech—you must be ready when opportunity strikes
- When to start job-seeking strategies—it's not when you think
- How to write a winning cover letter and résumé-even with zero work experience
- What never to say when asked, "What's your greatest weakness?"—don't make this fatal error
- Why you must tell stories—words tell, but stories sell!
- What hiring managers are really looking for in a candidate: essential insider tips from a hiring nurse manager

Here in your hands is the resource you need— all the best tips and topics in one place. You will learn how to compose a résumé designed to grab the recruiter's attention and land you an interview. You will be given the key elements needed for writing a cover letter or essay. You will be given all the tools you need to succeed in your job interviews. You will be an amazing nursing candidate—trust me!

The heart of this book for me is that I believe that there are many, many excellent nurses and nurses-to-be out there who are just an outstanding résumé or interview away from landing their dream job. Not just landing their dream job, but being compassionate, competent, caring nurses. That's who I want to reach with this book, by helping with my experience and expertise in career counseling.

Let's get started getting you a job so you can get started nursing!

1

Job Outlook

Always bear in mind that your own resolution to succeed is more important than any one thing.

—Abraham Lincoln

JOB MARKET FOR NEW GRADS

Is anyone else getting super frustrated with trying to apply for jobs? I've applied like over fifty times, but I feel like nobody's even looking twice at my application. How am I supposed to get that experience if no one is willing to give it? Sorry for the rant. Just wanted to see if I'm the only one and if anyone has found anything to work for them.

—*ASKED BY NEW GRADUATE NURSE RYAN*

Attempting to land a job is bewildering and frustrating for many new grad RNs. They are told time and time again that there's a shortage of nurses, but when they apply, their applications are turned down time and time again. This is when it's important to persevere and to strategically understand the job market.

NURSING SHORTAGE?

The fact is that nursing is currently one of the largest and fastest-growing occupations in the country. America's three million nurses make up the largest segment of the healthcare [1]workforce in the United States. Despite the growth, demand is predicted to exceed supply.

According to the Bureau of Labor Statistics,[1] 1.2 million vacancies will exist for registered nurses between 2014 and 2024. By 2025, some expect the shortfall to be larger than any other nurse shortage

---

1 U.S.Bureau of Labor Statistics. Occupational Outlook Handbook. Accessed April 2017 https://www.bls.gov/ooh/healthcare/registered-nurses.htm

experienced since the introduction of Medicare and Medicaid in the mid-1960s.

What are the reasons for the predicted nursing shortage? Aging and retiring baby boomers, healthcare legislation, and an emphasis on preventative care are the primary driving forces in this looming crisis. Today there are more Americans over the age of sixty-five than at any other time in US history. Between 2010 and 2030, nearly one in five Americans will be aged sixty-five and older. The need for healthcare professionals will be greater than ever.

While acute-care nurses will be needed, the healthcare landscape is shifting to the community. More services will be provided in outpatient settings. Advanced-practice RNs will be needed to fill the gap and serve as providers. Certified registered nurse anesthetists are leading the way in demand and income. Employment of CRNAs is predicted to grow 25 percent from 2012 to 2022, much faster than the average for all occupations. Nurses at all levels of preparation will be needed as never before.

NURSING SHORTAGE REDEFINED

In the face of such a critical shortage of nurses, why is it so difficult for a new grad to land a job? Sometimes even family members do not understand when a new grad is unable to immediately secure a position, and protest, "There's a nursing shortage, isn't there?" This only adds to the new grad's distress and sense of failure.

The reality is that a shortage of experienced nurses exists combined with a surplus of new graduate nurses. Hospitals need a balance of both experienced nurses and new graduate nurses to assure patient safety. It is frustrating for new grads to encounter job posting after job posting that specifies "experience required."

In addition, the "nursing shortage" is variable by region. In California, for example, there is a surplus of nurses in more desirable coastal areas like San Francisco and San Diego and a shortage of nurses in the less desirable rural areas.

> *Leslie lives in the San Francisco Bay Area. She had her hopes set on working L&D in a local prominent hospital. She eagerly kept checking and rechecking the status of her online application. After several weeks, she was finally informed, "We would like to advise you that your application does not meet our needs for the position at this time. This is not a reflection on your abilities; rather it is based*

on the lack of a match of relevant criteria with the information you provided. Please do not let this discourage you from applying for other or future opportunities with us."

Acute-care hospitals are not hiring many new grads in San Francisco. Because of the desirable location, employers can be very selective. This is true in many other desirable locations such as Hawaii. New graduate nurses in Hawaii are moving to the mainland to land their first nursing jobs. A new grad nurse who recently moved from Hawaii to Oregon said that entry-level nursing positions are very difficult to come by in Hawaii and that senior nurses are not leaving their hard-won positions.

Leslie must either apply at a less desirable location and relocate or apply to a less desirable job such as one in a skilled nursing facility (SNF) in her home area.

If this is your situation, consider relocating. The market for new grads is regional. Many new grads have found that if they are willing to relocate, they can land their first jobs and start gaining the experience they need. After one to two years, they will be an experienced nurse who has far more options and a pick of jobs.

Tip: If relocating, ask if travel reimbursement is offered. Some employers provide travel and relocation reimbursement, while others provide it only when asked. Be sure to keep your travel- and relocation-expense receipts for tax purposes.

SKILL ACQUISITION

The job market has shifted dramatically from the time when new grads could pick and choose. Some nurses still remember when new grads could get a job whenever and wherever they wanted. In today's market, hospitals can afford to be selective when it comes to hiring new grads. But as a result of nursing's past marketability and history, an entire generation of nurses has never had to learn the job-seeking skills that most college graduates must learn.

Many nurses hired in the 1980s reveal that they have never even had a proper interview. A nurse manager would approach them on the unit while they were in clinical rotation and say, "You're going to work here I hope, right?" The student nurse would smile and nod in assent. That was literally the extent of the hiring process—no résumé, no cover letter, and no interview. The old joke in nursing was that if you had a pulse, you were hired.

New graduate nurses today need job-seeking skills but many have never have acquired the skills. As a result, they are not prepared to compete in today's job market. How competitive is today's job market? Depending on location, extremely. There are many, many qualified applicants for each new grad position. My hospital recently received 304 applications for a nurse residency cohort with twenty-three available positions.

In fact, your best friends and classmates, Ashley and Kim, are now competing with you for the same job.

> *My application was for the (Cedar Sinai) new grad program. Most of us didn't have experience. They only took 60 of the 485 applicants to interview with HR. Then they narrowed it down to forty for the group interview and then twenty before the day was over, and now we are waiting to hear if we got one of the eight to ten positions they have available.*
>
> —*TIFFANY*

The eight to ten candidates who landed a position at this prestigious hospital in Los Angeles understood how to set themselves apart from the other 475 applicants. You will now learn how to do that as well.

Getting a job is your full-time job right now. It takes effort, commitment, and skills. New skills can be learned, but even with skills, you have to strategize in order to stand out.

By the end of this book, you will have the skills and strategies necessary for you to succeed. Even in today's competitive job market, savvy new graduate nurses and experienced nurses are landing the jobs they want every day—and you can be one of them!

1. United States Bureau of Labor, "Registered Nurses," *Occupational Outlook Handbook*, accessed April 2, 2017, https://www.bls.gov/ooh/healthcare/registered-nurses.htm.

2

Application Process

Only I can change my life. No one can do it for me.

—Carol Burnett

When you are applying to a job posting, you don't have the benefit of wowing the employer with your winning personality, engaging smile, and positive aura. You are limited to relying on the written or, more often, the electronic word.

If only they'd meet me in person, I'm sure they'd see what a great nurse I'd be! I know I could impress them, but I can't get past the application part. It's soooo frustrating.

—Jessica, NEW GRAD NURSE

You are screened not by your face-to-face presence and charm but by your ability to follow instructions. Your application must therefore be accurate, complete, and timely throughout the entire process. Careless mistakes are cause sufficient for your application to be rejected.

There is a belief by some that people who make careless mistakes and do not follow instructions on job applications make careless mistakes and do not follow instructions on the job. There are eagle-eyed human resource assistants waiting to toss your application into the do-not -call pile.

The point is that you can be the best nurse in the world but lose a job opportunity because you rushed or made mistakes in your application. Think of the application process as the employer's first impression of you. Put your best foot forward.

FOLLOW THE PROCESS

The nurse hiring process can be lengthy and complicated. Pay close attention to instructions at each step since you are being evaluated on your ability to follow them precisely. Do not assume that the employer will be flexible and make exceptions on your behalf if you do not follow instructions.

Alexandra lives on the West Coast and wants to work in Boston. The instructions were to "e-mail the application with all documents by 12:00 p.m. EST by January 4 to be considered for the spring program starting at the end of February."

Waiting until Friday, she forgets to adjust for the three hours' time difference and misses the opportunity. She is surprised when she calls and finds that they will not accept her late application and are not more flexible.

Allow yourself plenty of time for last minute, unforeseen delays or technical problems. Approach your job search with the same seriousness and focus as when you prepared for and took the NCLEX.

It's that important.

DON'T WAIT TO APPLY—YOU'LL BE LATE!

It's important to start your job search before you take the NCLEX and while you are still in school. Waiting until you graduate to start applying can delay your entry into a nursing residency by up to six months.

Many hospitals interview and hire nursing students into residencies that start a few months after they graduate with the contingency that they obtain their RN licenses before or during orientation.

The job posting will specify. Here are some examples:

- An RN license is required at time of hire.
- An RN license is not needed to apply for a position, but if an offer of employment is made, an RN license must be posted on the BON website before August.
- Once you have graduated and have a date scheduled for an NCLEX exam (or have already passed), please complete an online application for the RN position on our careers page that is most in line with your nursing career goals.

One major reason for getting a head start on your job search is that if you hit the one-year mark and have not landed a job, you are no longer eligible for most new grad residencies. Here's what happened to Brad:

> *I graduated from nursing school thirteen months ago. I took the summer off to take one last extended camping trip before starting work. I took my NCLEX two months ago.*

*I've been applying to new grad pro-
grams, and one of the recruiters
from a VA hospital told me that I'm
not considered a new grad anymore
since it's been a year that I graduated
from nursing school.*

—Brad, RN, NO LONGER A NEW GRAD

The clock starts ticking at the date of graduation.
Brad is neither a new grad nor an experienced
nurse, and that's an undesirable nonstatus to hold
when searching for a job. New grad status conveys
some benefits, such as eligibility to new grad residency programs, but new grad status only lasts for
about a year.

REQUIRED VERSUS PREFERRED

Some nurses are hesitant to apply to job postings
that specify "preferred" qualifications. Job postings
may say "preferred" or "required," as in:

- Preferred: Previous experience on a telemetry unit
- Required: BSN degree

In the first example, nurses who do not have experience on telemetry should apply, as it's not required
to have experience, just preferred. In the second

example, a BSN is required, so an applicant who doesn't hold a BSN does not meet stated qualifications and should not apply.

> *I got up my nerve and starting applying to jobs that said "BSN preferred," even though I don't have my BSN—and even to jobs that said six months' experience preferred but not required, so I would apply any way. Finally, I got an interview.*
>
> —*KIM, RN, NEW GRAD*

Even though the employer may *prefer* an applicant with experience, he or she will accept and consider applicants with no experience. You have nothing to lose by applying, and you may land a job.

> Tip: When employers specify "preferred," it means they anticipate that they may not receive enough qualified applicants and are hedging their bets. This works in your favor.

COMMON ERRORS

When uploading your résumé or cover letter, make sure you have updated the current date on the document. Also make sure you have updated the name of the hospital to which you are applying. It is easy to forget both of these things when you are applying to several facilities, but these can be fatal mistakes.

Do not name your file *résumé.docx*. Files so named will be lost in the receiver's computer folders. Name it with your first and last names like this: *Beth. hawkes.résumé.docx*.

Enlist friends to make sure they can open your document from various devices (mobile, laptop, and desktop).

REFERENCES AND LETTERS OF RECOMMENDATIONS

When selecting people to write letters of reference for you, choose carefully. Pick those who know you well and can speak to your skills, work habits, abilities, and character so that the letter will be authentic and not generic. Letters from present and past employers and educational institutions are preferable to letters from personal acquaintances.

Some employers ask applicants to submit references at the time of application. Some ask that they not be submitted until requested. Follow the instructions.

The following is from a large healthcare company: "The time needed to complete the reference-checking procedures sometimes causes a delay in our ability to extend contingent job offers. Therefore, we ask for references early in the job application process in an effort to reduce waiting times and provide a more efficient application experience. References are contacted only when a job seeker becomes a final candidate after interviewing. If you are in the interview process, you may alert the recruiter to any concerns you have about references."

Some employers ask new grads to submit one or two letters of recommendation specifically from clinical instructors. Why? Clinical instructors make credible references because they have observed your performance in clinical settings.

> *Try to get letters of recommendation from theory and clinical instructors after every class. It's much harder trying to get them after graduation. Ask for a general reference letter.*
>
> —*Ty, NURSING STUDENT*

Students, ask your clinical instructors for letters of recommendation immediately following your clinical rotations. Their memories and impressions of you will be strongest at that time. The recommendation letter will tend to be more impactful. Give your clinical instructor plenty of time to compose the letter. Clinical instructors can be inundated with multiple requests. Give your clinical instructor a list of accomplishments to help guide the letter and refresh his or her memory of your performance.

Note: Do not include "references available on request" on your résumé. It's no longer done, and you risk appearing dated. Employers requiring references will request them without a prompt from the applicant.

PREHIRE APPLICATION TESTS

Prehire application tests are used to assess the personality, skills, cognitive and attitudinal abilities of nursing candidates. In other cases, they are used post-hire to create independent learning plans for new grads.

While you can't study for a personality test, you can prepare. Watch for reverse wording of the same question, as you will be tested for consistency. Give similar answers to questions that ask the same thing. An example is: "I am conscientious and loyal," where you may answer "strongly agree" on a Likert scale. Later in the same test, you may be asked, "I am not conscientious and loyal," and you should answer "strongly disagree."

Such tests ask the same question or statement more than once to catch untruthful answers. Answering yes to both "I have never lied in my life" and "I once called in sick when I wasn't sick" signals dishonesty to the employer.

Be wary of questions or statements that test for socially undesirable but common behaviors and include absolutes such as "never" and "always." For example, "I am never angry" should not be answered "I strongly agree" since anger is a common human emotion.

Provide consistent, honest answers. Attempting to trick the test by giving answers you think the employer is looking for can alert employers to deception or exaggeration on your part. The tests test for inconsistency and report those scores as well. So just answer honestly, and be yourself.

If a question is confusing or vague, select the answer that best fits your personality or natural response.

PERSEVERE

> Hey, everybody! I just wanted to say
> I got my dream job—sixty-four appli-
> cations and only two interviews. But

what's cool is it happened, and it will happen for you too. Keep going; never give up. It will happen! I wish all of you the best in your future career path in nursing and want to thank you for all the support through these last couple of years. Seriously, thank you!

—*LISA, RN, NEW GRAD, FROM A SOCIAL MEDIA SITE*

It's true. You must stay the course. It's just like taking prerequisites for nursing school, and nursing school itself—half of succeeding in life is simply not quitting.

Perseverance may be the single most important factor in landing a job. Expect rejection (be realistic) but plan to persevere. Change your game plan but persevere. Adopt a multimodal approach and persevere. Never, ever give up. You will be rewarded.

Remember how far you've come. Trust the process. Let's get started with key insider tips and strategies.

3

Insider Tips and Strategies

I look for safe, clinically competent and loyal nurses who will be a good fit in my fast-paced emergency department.

—ASHLEY RODGERS, NURSING DIRECTOR

Y ou may have already realized that mass submissions of your résumé are not landing you a job. Mass submissions are the least effective method of landing a job and cannot be your only strategy. Here are some key tips to help you in your job search.

KNOW THE PLAYERS

Hospitals may seem like mammoth, intimidating, and impenetrable entities to the job seeker, but in truth, they are made up of real people with names, titles, and duties—people like you and me.

Having said that, not all people are equal when it comes to you and your job search. It's critical to know the players. The players are those who determine your employment future. The players have different roles from recruiter to office assistant to hiring manager, but each one has a key part to play once your application is submitted. Some players have more influence than others.

The Recruiter: The recruiter's job is to recruit and screen candidates. The recruiter may or may not be a nurse. To get past the recruiter, make sure you follow the organization's application directions to the letter and that your résumé is free of errors. Recruiters like to recruit candidates; it's their job to find qualified applicants. Often the recruiter can be a helpful source of information for you. Cultivating a relationship with a recruiter can be to your benefit.

Human Resources (HR): In many organizations, hospital-based recruiters work under the HR department but not always. HR has a major role in the hiring process, but HR does not hire you. You can dress up in your nicest outfit and pay a visit to HR, and it will likely do you no good. You will be greeted by smiles and someone saying, "We will call you." HR conducts background checks and verifies information.

The Nurse Manager: Nurse managers are the players who hire nurses. Ultimately, nurse managers hold the hiring power. It is nurse manager who decides which of the four applicants from a narrowed-down group of forty-five will land one of the openings on his or her nursing unit.

Lastly, there's the informal but influential advisory board to the nurse manager or the nurse manager's posse. This is tongue in cheek as there is no real advisory board, but nurse managers rely heavily on the opinions of charge nurses and respected staff, including certified nursing assistants (CNAs) and patient-care technicians (PCTs), when evaluating new staff for hire. This is because nurse managers look for a good fit for their units and rely on trusted staff to help them make that assessment. To summarize:

- Recruiters search for qualified applicants.
- Human resources verify applicants.
- Advisory boards influence nurse managers.
- Nurse managers hire applicants.

KNOW WHAT COUNTS

You are competing with many applicants who are equally qualified. All employers have methods of narrowing down multiple applications, and this is done before they ever meet you. Actually, it's done to determine if they are going to meet you.

At every facility, applications are evaluated by someone using some kind of metric or tool. This is how candidates are narrowed down to determine who will be offered a job interview. At my hospital, applications are scored via a point system by the director of our nurse residency program, my good friend Jamie. There are eight possible points:

- GPA > 3.75
- Employee referral
- Current employee
- Collaborative position with local college (hospital-sponsored seat)
- Essay/cover letter (up to three points)
- Community volunteer work

KNOW WHAT NURSE MANAGERS WANT

It's been said before, and it bears repeating. One of the best insider tips is that nurse managers look for a good fit for their nursing units. Nurse managers spend a lot of time and effort developing their staff, and they are very protective of their teams. They want to safeguard and preserve the culture on their units. They understand that one bad hire can change the dynamics of their entire group and nursing unit.

They are not looking for the person with the most certifications or the one who can explain the oxyhemoglobin disassociation curve. They can teach you ACLS and stroke alert and how to document, and they can train you to be a competent nurse. Knowledge alone is not sufficient to be a successful nurse.

While they cannot teach you how to be a good fit, they will judge whether you are one or not. They are forming impressions of you at each and every point of contact, from your cover letter, to your résumé, to your interview. You are being evaluated all along the way as to whether you are a good fit. You must be a good team player, loyal and authentic with high integrity.

The highest praise a manager can give after an interview is to turn to the other panel members, nod, and say, "I think they'd be a good fit."

> Tip: Find a way to put yourself in front of the players. You need face-to-face time to impress and stand out. There will be more creative strategies later about how to do this.

KNOW YOUR POTENTIAL EMPLOYER
Research your potential employer.

You've no doubt heard it said that you should research each potential employer and know the mission and values statement, but you may not have been told what it means to use the information in a savvy way.

> *Recently, Amanda came in for a panel interview. At one point, she rattled off the mission statement and then exclaimed that the hospital is Joint Commission (JC) accredited. It was somewhat out of context to the conversation and seemed contrived. When Amanda left, the Tele nurse manager rolled her eyes and said, "I'm soooo tired of applicants telling us about ourselves. I don't need one more person to tell me we are JC accredited."*

Amanda had done her homework, but she regurgitated the information in a manner that *focused on herself (showing how much she knows) rather than showing how she can help* meet the employer's needs. Evidently Amanda had been advised to "learn about the organization."

Instead of parroting the information, she could have asked a thoughtful question such as: "I understand that your organization does a lot of community work. Would there be opportunities for me to participate?"

Here are some practical and savvy examples of researching a prospective employer:

- If you know someone who works at the targeted facility, call that person and ask, "What's unique about the culture?" You may be surprised to hear, "We start morning huddles with prayer." Now you can reflect on this and speak to those values in your application process.
- Find out if they are magnet certified or on the magnet pathway. Magnet hospitals value education since a requisite number of staff has to be certified and hold bachelor's degrees. During your interview, you could highlight your future educational goals and ask questions about how they help with or provide continuing education.
- Magnet hospitals also have shared governance—a governing structure in which nurses participate. They want engaged nurses who will join committees. Can you see how that knowledge can help you be a good fit?
- Find out if they are stroke certified or an accredited chest-pain center. You could then

focus on your NIHSS stroke certification or express your interest in cardiac patients.

- Which electronic medical record (EMR) platform are they using: EPIC? Cerner? MediTech? Are they migrating to a new system? You will appear savvy if you know this, and it is even better if you can say you have had experience with the platform.
- What are their HCAHPs scores? All hospitals are working to improve their patient satisfaction scores since patient satisfaction is tied to reimbursement. Nurse managers are held responsible for meeting quality goals and improving HCAHPs.
- Have you had specialized communication training such as AIDET? This shows how you can help them achieve their patient satisfaction goals.
- What is their ethnic patient population breakdown? Are you fluent in a language used by many of their patients?

JOB POSTINGS

Hi, all—I'm just beginning my job search. I'm in the Bay Area. Please excuse my ignorance, but I'm not sure where to start. I'm doing Google searches (Indeed, etc.) and individual hospital websites. Is it true that most new grad jobs are posted at certain times of the year for a very short amount of time? Can anyone share some knowledge of when these are posted? Springtime? I can hardly find anything posted for any hospitals as far as an actual new grad program/ residency.

—NEWLY GRADUATED NURSE

When searching for job, it's important to use job boards, job search engines, word of mouth, and a variety of sites because no single site searches all job boards or employer sites. Sign up to receive alerts on job boards, but know that there can be a day or two lag between when the job is posted on the hospital's site and when it is posted on a job board.

Many hospitals have a narrow window of time for posting new grad job openings, some even forty-eight hours or less. Check selected hospital job postings regularly if not daily. You cannot predict when they will open applications for their next new grad residency, although many run two cohorts per year. Some hospitals open applications for a short window, and some have open application. Hospitals can change their posting patterns at any time depending on their needs at the time. Here's an example:

> Hospital A opened its application window four months before the residency start date. Their recruiter later discovered that neighboring Hospital B opened its application five months before the residency start date in order to be more competitive and offer jobs to the best and brightest applicants of the local graduating class. Now Hospital A is going to try an "always open" approach and evaluate how it works for their institution.

Either hospital can change its posting patterns at any time. By contrast, a large and prestigious hospital in Los Angeles runs a forty-eight-hour application window for new grads twice a year—period. If called, human resources does not reveal the upcoming open window dates. The point is that you must be vigilant in reviewing hospital postings. It's difficult, if not impossible, to predict when job openings will be posted.

Keep an Excel spreadsheet with names of facilities, passwords to their sites, dates, deadlines, and so on. When speaking to people, ask for their names. Note their names, the date, and the information they provided.

> Tip: Many new graduate nurses specify that they only want to work in intensive care, the emergency department, or labor and delivery. These specialty area requests narrow their chances. Indicate that you are open to working where there is a need. Most hospitals have open med surg positions. After a year or so, you can always apply to transfer to the specialty area of your choice. As an inside applicant, you will be given preferential consideration.

ELEVATOR SPEECH

You need an elevator speech. We all need an elevator speech. An elevator speech is a short, persuasive speech to tell others about you and to pique their interest in you. You should have your elevator speech polished and ready because you never know when an opportunity will present itself. Be prepared.

An elevator speech should:

- Be short. Sixty seconds, tops; thirty is better. Be succinct but impactful.
- Be memorable (personal examples help). Introduce yourself such as, "Hi, I'm Beth. B as in butterfly. Ha-ha." Silly? Maybe. But will they remember me? Yes!
- Be delivered energetically and enthusiastically.
- Be goal oriented (networking, job seeking).
- Tell them what you're passionate about.
- End with a call to action if appropriate to the situation.

An elevator speech can be modified for use at a meet and greet, any networking function, a conference, or a job fair. Here's an example of a very short elevator speech used at a job fair or conference. The goal here is to engage the recruiter in conversation and to spark his or her interest: "I'm Laura Lee. Nice to meet you. I'm a newly graduated nurse. I've been in school forever and can't wait to start my nursing career. I am passionate about pediatric nursing. Can you tell me more about what your hospital is looking for?" This is an example of projecting a confident, professional you. So few applicants are polished and professional that you will stand out by default.

MISSED OPPORTUNITY

I was recently chatting with Ashley, a nursing student who is graduating in two weeks and hopes to work in my hospital. We were standing in the hall outside the elevators when who should step out of the elevator but my good friend and nurse residency director, Jamie. I said, "Hi, Jamie. Hey, let me introduce you to Ashley. Ashley has just submitted her residency application. Ashley, meet Jamie. She's our residency director. You want to remember her name, ha-ha. It's J-A-M-I-E."

Ashley shyly extended a limp hand, looked downward, and said, "Hi." She missed a golden opportunity to make a lasting impression. There she was, face-to-face with the person who would put her application in either the reject pile or the keep pile, and she completely missed the opportunity to make herself memorable. Ashley was caught off guard, and her shyness took over. The way to avoid this is to be prepared. Compose an elevator speech now and start using it. You will be ready when the opportunity presents itself.

What could Ashley have done differently? Rewind: "Hi, Jamie. I'm so glad to meet you. I've heard such nice things about you from Jean, my clinical instructor. I've applied to your residency program, and I want you to know I am passionate about pediatrics. I want to work here because of the way your pediatrics program is growing. My son's pediatrician is Dr. Pal, and she practices here. She's told me several times how she prefers the nursing staff here at Happy Hospital." Or: "My name is Ashley Jenkins. I hope you'll take a second look at my application. Jamie, would it be OK if I call you later in the week to touch base?"

Notice that Ashley's elevator speech included a memorable example and ended with a call to action ("would it be OK if I call you later?").

PRACTICE, PRACTICE

The more you practice, the better. Practice out loud, not just in your thoughts. Without practice, you are apt to ramble, repeat yourself, or freeze. Practice in front of the mirror. Record yourself. Practice until you are comfortable.

I recently talked with another fourth-semester student, who started out very focused: *"Hi. I love it here; it feels like family. I want to work in L&D. I've loved it ever since I cared for my sister when she had a long recovery following a C-section."*

At first I was impressed, but then quickly I was not. Why? She didn't stop. I confess I soon tuned her out for two reasons.

- She is a soft talker, and her voice ebbed and flowed. We were in a noisy crowd of people, and it became too hard to keep asking, "What? Sorry?" Keep a strong, even pitch.
- She rambled. I quickly realized there were no structure and no end in sight as she repeated herself effusively.

Try using an elevator speech the next time someone asks, "What do you do?" and gauge that person's reaction. Build on his or her response and refine your speech. Use it with the next person. Repeat. At first you will feel uncomfortable. Being uncomfortable is a good thing because operating outside of your comfort zone means that you are acquiring new skills. Don't worry about sounding phony. Consider that TV personalities and celebrities use sound bites effectively all the time.

Delivery is everything. You need to be authentic, poised, and confident. Don't be rushed, too intense, or overly effusive. Practice so that you sound genuine, casual, and conversational. Practice does make perfect.

While you're at it, be mindful of your handshake. Make eye contact and offer a firm handshake along with a genuine, warm smile.

GET CONNECTED, STAY CONNECTED

> *Jake has recently graduated and talks to friends, relatives, and professors about looking for a nursing job. This steadily yields more advice and some more contacts. It turns out that Jake's neighbor's Rotary friend and golfing partner is CEO of the local hospital. His strategy is paying off.*

You are probably more connected than you know. Hospitals are large employers of all kinds of people. It is almost guaranteed you that if you start talking to any random person in your community, you could arrive at a connection at any hospital within a few degrees of separation.

Let everyone know you are looking for a job. This is not a time to be shy or self-effacing. Confident, connected people land jobs. Know that there are great things in store for you and they are just around the corner.

4

It's Not All about You

Strive not to be a success but rather to be of value.

—A*LBERT* E*INSTEIN*

CHANGE YOUR POINT OF VIEW

It's essential that you see things from a new and different point of view—the employer's point of view. The employer sees you (and hundreds just like you) as a new grad applicant—qualified, yes, but lacking experience. Being qualified is basic, and while being qualified is necessary, it does not set you apart. Basically, everyone you are competing with is qualified.

Lorelei couldn't understand why the CEO (and also her neighbor) at her local hospital was not particularly impressed with the fact that she had received top marks on a hand-washing poster board for her senior project. "He doesn't care about that," I told her (bluntly because she is my sister).

"He should," she exclaimed indignantly. "He should care. If only he understood how much infection would decrease and how that would translate into saving money."

> Lorelei couldn't get out of her student head. She wasn't going to get far clinging to her student mind-set and values, which also included listing details of each and every clinical rotation; that took up the top third (prime real estate) of her résumé. Lorelei needed to learn to think like an employer. In this instance, the CEO's most challenging problem at the time was reducing patient readmissions to avoid Medicare penalties—right or wrong, it was not hand washing.

Note: I am so proud of my sister, Lorelei. She has gone on to be a talented nurse leader in a large hospital, which is exactly what I expected of her.

THINK LIKE A BOSS

You must begin to think like an employer as you construct your résumé and stop thinking like a nursing student. Getting hired is largely a function of showing what you can do for the employer. Anticipate what they are looking for in an employee and show that you are a match. Employers want employees who will help them achieve their business goals, employees who are solutions to their problems.

> To quote Kyle Schmidt at bluepipes.com, *You're looking for information you can present as a problem, or potential problem, for which you are the solution. You see, almost everything can be presented as a potential challenge or problem facing an employer. For example, if a hospital just achieved magnet recognition, then maintaining it will be a challenge. The same goes for any award or recognition an employer has achieved. Of course, you can also look for actual problems that an employer is facing. For example, an employer may have a high employee turnover rate, or they may be in the process of attempting to achieve some goal or milestone, or they may be undergoing an EMR conversion in the near future.*

The winning equation is: Your Qualifications = Their Needs. If they are:

- Experiencing high turnover, they need loyal, committed employees.
- Magnet certified or on the magnet pathway, they need nurses who are motivated to further their education and professional development and participate in shared governance. You need to communicate that you are that committed, professional nurse.
- Struggling with their patient satisfaction scores, they need nurses with customer service skills.

What are their business goals? What are their problems? You need to know so that you can position yourself as not just a nurse who attended clinicals and passed the NCLEX but as an astute employee who will boost their HCAP scores and help meet their quality patient-care metrics.

Employers are looking for competent, dependable, reliable employees. They want nurses who are compassionate and safe practitioners with collaborative skills who are good team players. Smart hiring nurse managers look for candidates who display these characteristics and aspire to help them grow.

Remember, from now on, think like an employer. What are they looking for? What problems do they face? How can you be seen as a help to them?

5

Networking

No matter how technical the world gets, opportunities still happen through people.

—Carol Bush, The Social Nurse

Networking nets jobs. Professional networking is widely considered by many to be the most effective way of finding a job and even more so in challenging economic times. Some sources say up to 70 percent of jobs are acquired through networking. There's a reason why. It makes really good sense. If you were a hiring manager, you would prefer to hire someone known over someone unknown, right? We all would.

Many job opportunities are never posted or advertised but are only available by word of mouth. It's true that often it's not what you know but who you know. People like to help people they know and like, and that is the relational aspect of networking.

WHAT IS NETWORKING REALLY?

It's building, creating, and nurturing professional connections and relationships. It enables you to learn about job opportunities. According to Keith Carlson, master nurse networker, in his book *Savvy Networking for Nurses*, networking is not simply acquiring business cards and adding names to your LinkedIn account, it's developing relationships with people in the areas in which you are interested and staying in touch with them throughout your career. Networking is a mind-set of being ready and enlarging your professional circle.

Keith is so right. I would go so far as to say that, from my experience and in my career, networking is everything. You must embrace it. Successful networking takes ongoing nurturing of existing relationships and continual relationship building.

Let's explore some common networking myths.

NETWORKING MYTHS

Myth #1: Networking is for established nurse professionals, not me.

On the contrary, successful professional networking starts when you meet your first nursing professor or are assigned to your first preceptor. If you have friends who are starting school, do them a favor them and tell them that networking starts in first semester. If you are in a clinical setting, then you need to be networking.

Tip: Nursing is a small world. The nurse who precepted you in Hospital A may be a nurse manager in Hospital B by the time you graduate. Good thing you kept her or his contact information! Build your contacts and save phone numbers.

Myth #2: Networking is selling, and I don't like selling anything, much less myself.

In the working world, you have to put your best foot forward, make contacts, and sometimes promote yourself. Who is going to represent you if not you? It's not selling; it's more like wearing your best outfit to important functions.

Whether you acknowledge it or not, you have a brand; you *are* a brand, and you are constantly branding yourself. Denying that you are constantly messaging impressions of yourself to others is wishful thinking.

Myth #3: I'm not an extrovert, and you have to be an extrovert to network.

Not true at all. You have to be your authentic self. Contrary to what introverts believe and fear, networking doesn't mean gregariously flitting around the conference room, business card in hand. Networking is being genuinely interested in others and making connections. Introverts and extroverts both connect effectively with others, just in different ways. Effective networking is about connecting effectively.

LEVERAGE YOUR NETWORK

The people you already know—friends, family, neighbors, acquaintances, teachers, and former coworkers—are some of the most effective surprise resources for your job search. These people also have networks, and the people they know can lead to information about specific job openings that are not publicly posted or not yet posted.

You know more people than you realize.

- Go back and pay a visit to your *clinical instructors*. Ask for their help. Clinical instructors have strong connections to acute-care hospitals, and they have friends who are nurse managers.
- Likewise, ask your *preceptors* to put in a word for you. Stay in touch with them.

- Contact *classmates* of yours who already have a job. Ask them to put in a word to the nursing manager. Ask them for their hiring tips. How did they land their jobs?

Expand your network

- Participate in *online and social-media nursing communities*, groups, and forums. They provide support and information on job postings as well as tips.

  Facebook has entire pages/groups devoted to new grads who are searching for jobs by geographical region. They exchange helpful information daily. Often they share about hospitals offering jobs before the job postings hit the job boards, or they give tips or examples of how their interviews went. At the very least, these groups can be a great support.

- Attend *job fairs and conferences*. You never know who you'll meet or what contacts you'll make.
- Join LinkedIn to connect with other nurses and recruiters. Grow your LinkedIn network. After meeting someone at a conference or elsewhere, send the individual a personalized invitation to connect on LinkedIn.

- Get out in your community. Go to the farmer's market. Go to the *gym* regularly. Many nurses go right before or after their shifts; go at that time and talk with them. The same applies for *church* if you attend. Be visible.

You must continuously make new contacts and nurture old contacts. To develop new contacts, join student, community, or professional organizations.

OPPORTUNITY STRIKES

Here's a great example:

> *I was babysitting and chatting with the children's father when they got home. He asked me about nursing school and my graduation, which was coming up shortly. He asked me what specialty I wanted to work in. I told him I wanted to work in oncology. He asked me if I'd applied to Hospital A, and I said, "Oh, no, they don't have an oncology service." He said he was pretty sure they did, and I corrected him again, repeating that I didn't think they had any oncology jobs and that I hadn't even bothered to apply there.*

Then I said jokingly, "Do you have some kind of insider information?"

With a smile, he said, "Well, I'm the CEO of the hospital, and I know for a fact that we are looking for oncology nurses. I think you should apply for a job in the new unit oncology unit we're opening." I could have died! I was so embarrassed. Here I was babysitting for him, and I had no idea he was the CEO of the hospital; how did I not know that?

So I applied and got an interview right away. Then I got the job! Whoot!

—As SEEN ON A SOCIAL-MEDIA SITE

Without a doubt, the CEO who entrusted his children to this nurse was impressed enough to put in a word for her at his hospital.

EMPLOYEE REFERRALS

Hospital employee referral programs are among the most aggressive in the country. They typically offer generous employee referral bonuses, which incentivize their employees to make referrals.

Granted, the bonuses are primarily given for experienced nurses, but an employee referral attached to your application can tip the odds in your favor.

> Tip: As a new grad, be wary of organizations that offer sign-on bonuses to new graduate nurses. This can be an indicator that they are unable to retain nurses and are desperate. This can be due to poor and unsafe working conditions such as extremely short orientation or high nurse–patient ratios. Reputable hospitals do not typically offer sign-on bonuses to new grads in today's market.

People around you see more in you than you see in yourself. Believe them when they tell you how wonderful you are. It's true. You are unique and wonderful

6

Certifications

I'm on the edge…of glory!

—Lady Gaga

Amanda graduated six months ago and is still trying hard to land a job. Her friends are urging her to obtain as many nursing certifications as possible in order to appear more marketable. Amanda knows that most of these courses are expensive, and on top of the course fee, she will have to purchase a pricey textbook. There are many companies out there targeting new nurses like Amanda with educational offerings, and she wants to spend her money and her time wisely.

Do certifications for new grad nurses boost résumés? Or do they just break your pocketbook? Here's what you need to know and how not to get conned.

Many new grads are spending good money and a lot of time obtaining multiple certifications such as ACLS, PALS, and so on. As a result, amassing certifications has become de rigueur. This trend did not start with employers but with desperate new graduate nurses.

Hiring managers understand that while accumulating certifications does show initiative, it does not convey expertise. They are not as impressed as you may hope. Employers are not looking for expertise in new grads because new grads do not have experience. Training without clinical experience/application is simply didactic knowledge.

If an ACLS is *required* for the job, the employer will typically provide the class for free and pay for your two-day attendance: "Must possess and maintain a current PALS and ACLS certificate or obtain within six months of hire."

Some businesses are even taking advantage of new grads by bundling and selling courses such as pharmacology and CPR/BLS. You already had pharmacology in school, so think twice before putting out money to take another course.

Take a balanced approach. Do maintain your American Heart Association (AHA) healthcare provider CPR/BLS. Make sure it's a healthcare provider course and provider card.

CERTIFICATIONS FOR NEW GRAD NURSES

Take only AHA courses for pediatric life support (PALS), basic life support (BLS), and advanced cardiac life support (ACLS). There are companies that offer 100 percent online courses, and that is a dead give-away that they are not AHA affiliated. AHA always requires a live skills check before issuing a provider card. The AHA and AAP do not endorse, nor are they affiliated with, *any* fully online certification program. Here are the pros and cons of taking courses on your own to boost your resume.

BASIC LIFE SUPPORT (BLS)

BLS is required for all nurses. Never, ever let it lapse as it's a professional expectation to maintain your BLS.

Always:

- Take BLS from an American Heart Association (AHA) instructor (not an AHA copycat).
- Take the AHA healthcare provider courses (not a nonhealthcare provider course and not hands-only BLS).

BLS renewal courses are four hours long and can cost under fifty dollars, but costs vary according to the instructor/company. AHA does not dictate costs. A two-year provider card is issued.

Pros: Professional requirement
Cons: None

ECG COURSES

Unlike ACLS, PALS, and National Institute of Health stroke scale (NIHSS) certifications, electrocardiography (ECG) courses are not standardized. Anyone can offer an ECG course, and the length may vary from a few hours to a few weeks. At the end of the course, you may be issued a certificate of completion, but these are homegrown and do not carry an expiration date or convey a provider status.

Therefore, hospitals put little stock in an ECG certificate of completion and instead test for competency by administering their own basic arrhythmia competency test. Basic arrhythmia competency is required for ICU, step-down, tele, and ED nurses. Many hospitals also require it for L&D (to recover a C-section) and med surg (remote tele) nurses.

The value in taking an ECG course is that you it prepares you to take and pass the basic arrhythmia competency test.

Pros: Very good for professional development; prepares the learner to pass basic arrhythmia competency.

Cons: If required for your job, the employer will provide this course for free, and most will pay you to attend.

ADVANCED CARDIOVASCULAR LIFE-SUPPORT COURSE (ACLS)

ACLS is an AHA course that trains healthcare providers to participate in or manage a code. ACLS is ten to twelve hours long and is generally required for ED and ICU, as well as tele, step-down, and sometimes med surg nurses, depending on the organization.

A prior understanding of basic arrhythmia is important as you will be expected to identify rhythms. The course is interactive with scenarios and simulations. ACLS courses can cost around $150, but costs vary according to the instructor/company. AHA does not dictate costs. A two-year provider card is issued.

Pros: Shows initiative.

Cons: If required for your job, the employer will provide this course for free, and most will pay you to attend. ACLS skills are better learned once you have attended a few codes and have some clinical context to build on.

NATIONAL INSTITUTES OF HEALTH STROKE SCALE (NIHSS)

NIHSS is offered by the National Stroke Association. It prepares learners to assess a stroke patient using video scenarios and to rate the stroke severity on a standardized scale. Offered in a self-paced, online training format, the course is free. The certificate is good for two years.

Pros: Shows initiative and is seen as a value by stroke-certified organizations; good for professional development and knowledge.
Cons: If required for your job, the employer will provide this course for free, and most will pay you to attend.

TRAUMA NURSING CORE COURSE (TNCC)

This sixteen- or twenty-hour intensive course was developed by the Emergency Nurses Association (ENA) and prepares the learner to manage trauma patients.

Not all EDs are trauma centers, and nurses in non-trauma EDs are not required to have their TNCC. TNCC courses can cost around three hundred dollars, including textbook, but cost varies by instructor/company. A four-year provider card is issued.

Pros: Shows initiative and may be helpful for an ED position.

Cons: Specific to trauma and trauma EDs only. If required for your job, the employer will provide this course for free, and most will pay you to attend.

EMERGENCY NURSING PEDIATRIC COURSE (ENPC)

This sixteen-hour comprehensive course was developed by the ENA. It provides ED nurses with the knowledge and skills to care for pediatric patients. ENPC courses can cost around three hundred dollars, including textbook, but cost varies by instructor/company. A four-year provider card is issued.

Pros: Shows initiative and may be helpful for an ED position.

Cons: Specific to EDs. If required for your job, the employer will provide this course for free, and most will pay you to attend.

PEDIATRIC ADVANCED LIFE-SUPPORT COURSE (PALS)

The fourteen-hour AHA PALS course prepares pediatric nurses to resuscitate and stabilize infants and children experiencing cardiopulmonary arrest. PALS skills, like ACLS skills, are better learned once you have attended a few codes and have some clinical context. PALS is often required for ED, ICU, and pediatric nurses. PALS courses can cost around $140, but costs vary according to the instructor/company. AHA does not dictate costs. A two-year provider card is issued.

Pros: Shows initiative and may be helpful for a position working with pediatric patients.
Cons: If required for your job, the employer will provide this course for free, and most will pay you to attend.

NEONATAL RESUSCITATION PROGRAM (NRP)

NRP is based on the American Academy of Pediatrics (AAP) and AHA guidelines for cardiopulmonary resuscitation and emergency cardiovascular care of the neonate and trains the learner for emergency care and resuscitation of the newborn. NRP courses are offered as a blend of self-study, online exam, and classroom skills/simulation portion.

The simulation portion is about four hours long. NRP courses can cost around $140, but costs vary according to the instructor/company. It may be required for L&D and NICU nurses, depending on the facility. A two-year provider card is issued.

Pros: Shows initiative and may be helpful for a position working with neonates.

Cons: If required for your job, the employer will provide this course for free, and most will pay you to attend.

STABLE PROGRAM

STABLE is a neonatal program that focuses on stabilizing newborns. STABLE stands for the six assessment parameters taught in the course: sugar, temperature, airway, blood pressure, lab work, and emotional support. It's an eight-hour class and can cost around $150, including textbook, but costs vary according to the instructor/company. A completion card is good for two years.

Pros: Shows initiative and may be helpful for a position working with newborns.

Cons: If required for your job, the employer will provide this course for free, and most will pay you to attend.

FINAL TIPS ON CERTIFICATIONS FOR NEW GRAD NURSES

Don't spend more than you can afford, and compare prices. Some companies charge more than others. Don't take anything unnecessary. For example, taking an IV certification course in CA is not necessary as IV certification is not required. IV start skills are taught in nursing school.

Watch out for poorly defined courses and consider why you should take a course that you already took in nursing school. Think twice about bundled courses such as ECG and pharmacology when what you really want to learn is ECG.

No one loves ambivalence and feeling unsettled-but this too, shall pass.

7

Tips for Student Nurses

Thank a student today...for choosing nursing. They are the future of our profession!

—*Donna Cardillo, RN, the Career Guru at Nurse.com*

I am so glad you are reading this if you are a nursing student. I am especially fond of nursing students and new nurses.

You are determined and goal oriented to have gotten as far as you have. Bravo! These characteristics will help immensely in your job search. Whether it's your first semester or your last, congratulations on your career choice.

When you're a student, you live in an insulated bubble where your entire world revolves around and is consumed by your grades, your next paper that's due, or your looming end-of-semester exam. It's easy to lose perspective and sight of everything else when you're in this long tunnel called nursing school.

The reason you're in a nursing program is to be a nurse. It's a mistake to think that you don't have to start thinking about your job search until after you graduate. The statistics about landing a job are not especially favorable for new graduate nurses, but the odds can be in your favor by strategizing now while you're still in nursing school.

MIND-SET OF A SUCCESSFUL RN

Right now, chances are that you see yourself as a student or perhaps as a desperate new grad. Wait. Take a step back—and look forward. Visualize yourself as a working RN and a sought-after commodity.

This gives you the confidence and initiative to launch your hiring plan. Be a confident you. The organization needs you; they just don't know it yet. Reframing your thinking and following the next nine steps will bring you opportunities.

START NOW

Strategizing to land your first nursing job starts now. Preferably it started in the first semester, but it is never too late to start planning. Think of the other students in your class. Chances are they see themselves as just that—students. Your study partner, Alexis, may only see as far ahead as the next care plan or maybe the upcoming neuro test. Diagnosis: tunnel vision.

Unlike your peers, you must never lose sight of the ultimate goal, which is to be a practicing RN, which means getting hired, which brings us back full circle to early strategizing.

KNOW WHO'S WHO

If you were asked right now who does the hiring of nurses in the hospitals, would you know the answer? Nurse managers, that's who—not human resources or nurse recruiters, although both are involved in the process. The nurse manager has the final say. Know who holds the hiring power. This understanding can help you right now—today—to land a job in the future.

It's easy for a student doing a clinical rotation on a nursing unit to be completely unaware of who's who, organization wise. Everyone looks the same in their lab coats or business attire, right? Besides, you're not an employee; you're a student. You're not motivated to learn the org chart; you've never even seen it, and the primary authority figure on *your* radar is your clinical instructor.

This is not to say you must learn the org chart, but as a job seeker, you need to learn who the nurse managers are by their names and by their departments. Think of it as homework on your next shift during your clinical rotation. It's that important to your future.

Nurse manager: She or he is the one who must be impressed. Keep in mind that nurse managers are busy people and seek the counsel of their advisory councils when making hiring decisions. Advisory councils are comprised of charge nurses, select trusted nursing staff (which includes nursing assistants and PCTs as well as RNs), and other nurse managers—all of which means that you have plenty of people to impress during your clinical rotations and lots of opportunity to do so.

WORK AS A NURSING ASSISTANT OR PCT

If at all possible, work as a certified nursing assistant (CNA) or patient-care technician (PCT) in the hospital you plan to apply at when you graduate. Many hospitals that require certified nursing assistants accept first-year nursing students as having had equivalent training. Work during summers, school breaks, and holidays. This is the number-one thing you can do to help secure a job when you graduate, and not because you have CNA or PCT experience per se. It's because they've had time to see you and your work ethic in action, unlike the other job candidates.

All things being equal, employers will hire a known applicant over an unknown applicant. When you work as a CNA or PCT, nurse managers know you, staff members have your back, and it's all around really, really beneficial for getting hired as a new grad. It goes without saying that you have been a reliable, hardworking, team-playing worker extraordinaire during your audition—I mean tenure—as a nursing assistant..

Nursing students who work as CNAs or PCTs have home field advantage. Voila! By doing so, you have made yourself a no-brainer hire for the nurse manager.

As a matter of fact, he or she will love you for making his or her hiring job easier. By hiring you, he or she has reduced his or her risk.

The nurse manager already knows that you fit in and that you deliver outstanding patient care. It's a beautiful win-win situation.

BE A SUPERSTAR

Clinical rotations are a job seeker's dream. In what other career do you get a chance to see and be seen time and time again before you apply for a job? Meet and impress the nurse managers or charge nurse during clinical rotations.

How do you do that? Look for opportunities; they will present themselves while you are in the hospital.

It doesn't matter that you're not on your dream unit. Hate step down? No worries. Later on, when you apply to work in the emergency department (ED), Stephanie, the step-down unit manager, will speak favorably of you to her BFF, Jessica, the ED unit manager. Jessica *will* snap you up.

WRITE A NOTE TO THE MANAGER

Write a note to the nurse manager after your clinical rotation. By write, I mean use a pen, and by note, I mean paper and envelope. Here's an example: "I learned so much during my clinical rotation on your unit. The staff was so supportive and helpful, especially Beth Hawkes. This is exactly the kind of nursing team I'd like to be a part of someday. Thank you for the experience" or a semblance thereof. Sign your name prominently. Stop by a week or so later to see if he or she got your note. Wait! There it is, pinned on the wall above the nurse manager's desk because everyone appreciates a personalized and handwritten note.

You have set yourself apart because very few nursing students will do this.

> Tip: Make sure your name is legible. You want them to remember your name.

VOLUNTEER

Get involved in community health events. This is a must so that you can add these volunteering experiences to your résumé. It's also an opportunity to learn how gratifying it is to give back and to start a lifetime of volunteering.

Some nursing programs arrange for their students to measure blood pressures or perform finger sticks at the county fair or at other community events. Pursue any such opportunities to volunteer. Attend church camp and shadow the camp nurse. Search online to become aware of community events and opportunities. In your nursing class, serve as an officer if possible. Mentor or tutor another student, perhaps a prenursing student struggling with chemistry.

When job candidates are running neck in neck, the tie breaker can come down to points awarded for community involvement and volunteering. I've seen this happen. Did I say points? Yes. Applicants are often graded on a point system, and candidates who volunteer are awarded extra points.

NETWORK. NETWORK. NETWORK.

Network, network! All things being equal, the person who is known will get the job over the person who is not known. There is no bad networking except for no networking.

Attend local conferences/CE events. Join the local chapter of the National Student Nursing Association (NSNA). This is good for résumé building as it shows a commitment to professional development.

Form relationships with your preceptors and keep in touch with them. When you graduate, you can contact them and ask them to give you a referral. You never know which former preceptor will go on to become a hiring manager. Reach out to the students who are in the graduating class ahead of you. They will graduate sooner than you, and many will be employed by the time you graduate. You can contact them to learn about job opportunities and to ask if one would serve as your job-searching mentor.

Using some of these ideas will undoubtedly help you think of your own creative strategies as well.

8

Standout Résumés

The difference between ordinary and extraordinary is that little extra.

—JIMMY JOHNSON

Your résumé can be your most effective marketing tool, or it can be a career obituary. When applicants are sending out multiple résumés and not landing interviews, the culprit is the résumé. In this chapter, you will learn how to make your résumé stand out from others. You will learn how to craft a winning résumé even when you are new to the field.

Ashley graduated six months and forty-two résumés ago without yet landing a single interview. Discouraged and depressed, she strongly considered giving up, but with a strategic revamp of her résumé, she landed her dream job in a pediatric acute-care unit.

The problem with Ashley's résumé was that it was exactly like the dozens of other new grad résumés that recruiters see every day. There was nothing to set it apart. She did not know how to make her résumé stand out from all the other ones from equally qualified but inexperienced applicants. In fact, Ashley herself thought she wasn't such a great candidate. She was actually a great candidate, but she needed to believe it and for her résumé to illustrate it.

How important is your résumé? Extremely.

- You have roughly six seconds to capture their attention.
- It's often the one and only chance you have to secure an interview.
- There are no do-overs once submitted.
- It's the first impression your potential employer has of you. First impressions are lasting and impactful.

It may seem evident that the purpose of a résumé is to land an interview, but résumés are commonly written as if the purpose is to use as many overused and tiresome clichés as possible.

A résumé is more than a laundry list of experiences; when effective, it's a compelling snapshot of *you*. If it's sufficiently compelling, you'll get the call for an interview.

Given that the purpose of your résumé is to answer the question "Why should we interview *you*?" it follows that everything you choose to include in your résumé should answer that question.

A common example of something that does not answer the question "Why should we interview *you*?" is a lengthy description of clinical hours. All qualified applicants attended and passed clinical rotations, so it only serves to show that you are like everyone else and that you have a student mind-set, not an employer's mind-set.

FORMATTING RULES YOU MUST FOLLOW

So now you know that you have only six to ten seconds to capture their inerest. Want to buy an additional six seconds? Your résumé must have visual appeal. Visual appeal causes the recruiter's eyes to linger on your résumé because it holds visual interest and provides visual rest.

Steve turned in a résumé with long, dense blocks of text and very little white space. There were no bullet points to break up and highlight the information. He wasn't getting any responses. He then reformatted it using the following suggestions. Within two weeks, he had two calls for interviews, and he had not changed the content.

White space and chunking is important for visual appeal. Lack of white space and long, dense paragraphs negate good content. There should be five to seven lines per paragraph and then a line break (white space) and repeat. This provides a needed respite for the eye and brain.

Your résumé should be consistent and pleasing in choice of font sizes and weights. The safest is to use one font type for the headers and the same font type for the body text. For example, use Times New Roman 12-point font for the text and Times New Roman 14-point font in bold for the header. Headers should be congruent in importance. Consistency aids in comprehension.

Bullet points aid in readability and guide the reader, but use bullets in a consistent manner. Bullets would provide a reader-friendly way to list accomplishments, for example, and to highlight important information.

Résumés must be mistake free. When résumés contain careless errors, it can be viewed as a predictor of carelessness on the job. When uploading a résumé into an ATS, make sure the date is updated. Common mistakes include having the wrong name of a hospital or facility. I recently saw a résumé with a date of 2027. Watch out for spelling errors not caught by spell check, such as "there" and"their".

It is a truism that errors are seen only after clicking send. So when you're finished composing your résumé, let it sit for a couple of days. When you pick it up, you will immediately see room for improvement.

Submit your completed résumé to several different eagle-eyed people for editing. In the print business, it is standard to have seven different people edit print copy. That is why you never see errors in *Time* or *People* magazines.

- Use a basic font such as Times New Roman, twelve point font.
- Avoid clever or artistic fonts, multiple fonts, graphics, or distracting colors.
- Use heavyweight, high-quality paper for résumés that you will take in your portfolio to an interview.
- Keep your résumé to one to two pages in length. One is best for entry-level workers.

VERBS AND TENSE

Every word should be carefully chosen. Use strong action verbs such as "developed," "achieved," "completed," "created," "attained," "initiated," and "exceeded." For example, instead of "helped on a project," say "coordinated project activities," and instead of "responsible for" (passive and weak), say "managed." Use a thesaurus or simply Google synonyms to expand your vocabulary repertoire. Your résumé will stand out.

Maintain the same tense and voice throughout, for example, first person and past or present tense. Do not use "I" or "my" even though you are writing in the first person.

KEYWORDS

Your résumé should mirror the values and culture of the organization. How do you do that? Use industry keywords from the job posting for your skills. Many organizations use keyword-scanning software to screen résumés. Have the job description in front of you as you compose your résumé.

Here's an example from a job posting: "Demonstrates leadership, effective communication, and excellent critical thinking skills. Join our team of compassionate and passionate healthcare professionals who are committed to the well-being of our patients and provide patient care based on competence, professional expertise, knowledge, and evidence-based practice." In your résumé, under clinical experience, you can highlight that your senior practicum project was on evidence-based practice for central line management. The keyword "evidence-based practice" will show in a keyword scan. In this instance, you are choosing to highlight evidence-based practice because the employer focused on it.

Note that you can use synonyms for keywords as ATS software is programmed to recognize constructs of the term.

AVOID CLICHÉS

A very common error is overly wordy résumés. It is easier to write long than to write short as short requires the skill of brevity. Résumés packed with tired phrases, buzzwords, and clichés do not add value and do not help you to stand out. In fact, they work against you in your quest to stand out.

Everyone is motivated and detail oriented, and by the time the recruiter has read "motivated and detail oriented" twenty times in one morning, it is simply annoying white noise. Avoid clichés such as "forward thinking," "change agent," "innovative," and "self-starter."

Can you put actual examples on a résumé? Yes. It's far better to use examples that illustrate qualities. Examples are remembered. Clichés are not. Consider "motivated, forward-thinking, detail-oriented individual" versus "initiated no-pass zone among colleagues in clinical rotation to answer call lights in a shorter time to improve patient safety and satisfaction."

The first example with its clump of clichés says nothing. The second example says you are patient-centered and forward thinking in your practice. Trust me, the second example would make any hiring nurse manager sit up straight in his or her chair and reach for the phone to call you.

CATEGORY SEQUENCING

Contrary to what you may have been taught, a résumé doesn't have to be in any preordained, chronological order. It can have the headers or categories you choose in the order you decide. It's your strategically designed résumé.

There are many good formats. People debate the dos and don'ts. But all agree that a poorly constructed résumé is likely to be put aside.

Résumé templates are an option but can be difficult to modify with preformatted columns and text boxes. In addition, recruiters instantly recognize the standard, canned Microsoft résumé templates.

Remember that the top one-third of your résumé is prime real estate. Top load the items you want the employer to see first, such as your necessary qualifications, RN license, date of graduation or NCLEX, BLS, and other certifications.

Here's one way for a new grad with limited work experience to sequence his or her categories:

- Contact information
- Objective statement/personal summary (optional)
- Qualifications, certifications, and education
- Professional skills
- Work experience
- Volunteer experience
- Professional affiliations (such as nursing organizations)

From this outline, you can change the order and customize/add categories such as an objective statement, honors, achievements, and professional affiliations (pick or create a headline/category that best highlights your accomplishments).

CUSTOMIZING

One of the best strategies is to individualize your résumé to each potential employer. This makes your résumé employer focused and not applicant focused. Winning résumés are not about you so much as about your targeted employer. If you are applying to five different facilities, you need five customized versions of your résumé (see Know Your Employer in chapter 1). For example, because you have done your research, you know which computer system they are using and can speak to your experience and proficiency with the system.

Never submit a résumé until you have performed due diligence in finding out about the hospital or company, what they stand for, and what they believe. Above all, they are looking for that person who is going to be a good fit.

Contact Information

If your e-mail address is zombiegirl@hotmail, get another one for professional contact information. Provide a phone number that won't be answered by children and has a professional-sounding recorded answering message. You can easily get a Gmail account dedicated for job searching and even a phone number. Add your LinkedIn contact information to your résumé if you have a LinkedIn profile.

Tip: Having a LinkedIn profile is recommended as it adds a level of professionalism and helps you to stand out.

OPTIONAL: OBJECTIVES/SUMMARY STATEMENTS

Personal summaries are preferable for experienced workers, while objective statements are fine for the entry-level applicant, but both are acceptable.

They are both optional because in the case of a new grad, there's not much in the way of a professional summary, and in all cases, it's evident that you are seeking a position. If used, this portion goes at the top. Whether you use objectives or summaries (your choice), keep it brief—fifty words or less, straightforward, and succinct.

Do not write complete sentences for objectives. Simple fragment statements are impactful. For example, compare "To obtain a position as a registered nurse with opportunities for professional development while providing excellent healthcare and customer service utilizing clinical skills, critical thinking, and evidence-based practice in conjunction with management, leadership, and organizational skills from previous professional experience" to this: "Energetic and compassionate new grad nurse seeking nursing position at Happy Pediatric Hospital."

The problem with the first example (a real-life example) is that it adds words without adding value. Watch out for this common tendency toward wordiness and fluffery.

QUALIFICATIONS, CERTIFICATIONS, AND EDUCATION

This section should be brief and not take up too much real estate on your résumé. Include your RN credential, relevant certifications (BLS, ACLS), and education.

Graduation date and school are all you need under education. Do not include a list of clinical rotations unless one of the rotations was at the hospital you're applying at, you did a senior practicum in a specialty area, or you have another strategic reason for inclusion.

Lengthy and wordy descriptions of your clinical hours are painful to read and do not set you apart. It is a given that you attended school and performed the requisite clinical hours in the requisite clinical settings. Likewise, do not include a list of duties.

Tiffany carefully enumerated all of her duties: "administered meds, provided patient care, obtained vitals," and so on.

You are not going to be interviewed based on a list of duties you performed in school. When you think like an employer, these are meaningless. Every new grad has administered meds and provided patient care. These are a given and do not answer the question "Why should we interview *you?*"

Do not include high-school information on a professional application unless instructed to do so. Include your GPA only if sets you apart; greater than 3.75 is a guideline. If your GPA is 3.25, there is no benefit in highlighting it unless asked.

YOU HAVE SKILLS

Note that in the following example, the category for professional skills is listed before work experience. This is an option for the candidate whose skills may be more impressive than his or her employment history.

WHAT ARE HARD SKILLS AND SOFT SKILLS?

Include hard skills *if they help you to stand out and are relevant to the position.* An example is experience with Cerner if they use Cerner or Epic if they use Epic. Hard skills are teachable skills.

Soft skills are transferable skills you've gained during school, extracurricular activities, volunteering, or in previous non-nursing jobs. Harder to quantify, soft skills are less tangible and are often interpersonal. Soft skills include those such as AIDET or other customer-satisfaction training, Toastmaster speaking skills, and team leading.

Soft skills set you apart. Employers look for candidates with strong soft skills because they are indicators of success on the job.

WORDS TELL, STORIES SELL

Give examples of your identified soft skills and personal characteristics. *Examples are remembered.* Were you ever selected as employee of the month (people person)? Do you have a perfect attendance record at school or work (reliable)? Did you study abroad? Do you know a second language? Have you supervised others? Are you composed under stress?

You may think that working is not relevant to working as a nurse, but holding a job for any respectable length of time shows reliability.

Did you tutor other students in school (helpful)? Did you sell Rodan cosmetics? Working for yourself shows a great deal of initiative and organizational ability.

Have you served in roles at church, taught in the nursery, or led a group study? Have you helped plan a retreat? All of these experiences have garnered you transferable skills.

WORK HISTORY

Work history is listed in reverse chronological order. Be prepared to explain any gaps in employment. That's one of the first things an experienced hiring manager looks for. Gaps can indicate unreliability and must be accounted for in a positive manner.

Don't list positions more than fifteen years old unless you held executive positions.

VOLUNTEER

If you have volunteer experience, this is worth putting in its own category. All things being equal, the candidate with volunteer experience can often be the one who lands the job.

CRITIQUE

Finally, look over your résumé with a new eye. Imagine that you are reading it for the first time—as a potential employer. Again, every single item included in your résumé should answer the question "Why should we interview *you?*"

CHECKLIST/SUMMARY

- Have you done your research on the facility?
- Did several people review your résumé?
- Is it succinct and easy to read?
- Is your contact information accurate and professional?
- Does your résumé answer the question "Why should we interview *you?*" throughout?

CREATIVE STRATEGIES

A creative strategy for a résumé is the use of humor. It's risky and not for everyone because humor can backfire or not translate well and is dependent on the receiver.

But if it succeeds, it sets you apart. An example is adding "Loves Nutella" Another creative strategy is to include a hobby. Many sources say not to, but, again, if you teach skydiving, the interest you garner may justify the risk.

TESTIMONIALS

OK, so I got the job. I rocked my résumé following your tips.

—RODNEY

Just looked over my résumé. It was like a poorly written epic novel, too wordy, painful, and unnecessary.

—STEPHANIE, RIGHT BEFORE SHE REVISED HER RÉSUMÉ AND WAS HIRED AS AN INFUSION SPECIALIST

Be extraordinary—because you are.

Nathan Smith

Home: 555-123-9876 Cell: 555-777-1212 **nathan-nurse@gmail.com**

Objective
Top-performing senior nursing student seeking new grad residency position at Happy Hospital

Licensure and Certification
BLS for Healthcare Providers, American Heart Association (AHA)

Advanced Cardiac Life Support (ACLS)

Certified Nursing Assistant #34522

Education
Cal State University TriCity: Los Angeles, CA *Expected graduation: May 2018*

Bachelor of Science in Nursing GPA 3.95

Professional Skills
Nursing Assistant

- Proficient in EHR documentation in Epic, Cerner, and MediTech

- Practices purposeful hourly patient rounding
- Named Employee of the Year by coworkers 2016
- Selected by nurse manager to orient new nursing assistants
- Proficient in conversational Spanish
- Follows up on all patient requests and checks back to see if their needs have been met
- Prioritizes patient safety by immediately reporting abnormal vital signs to RN
- Successful in mobilizing patients who need extra encouragement

Waiter

- Regularly resolved customer complaints to their satisfaction
- Anticipated and prioritized customer requests
- Coordinated with kitchen staff to provide service recovery when needed
- Consistently received highest tips
- Awarded one-year perfect attendance 2016

Volunteer Experience
LA County Pediatric Vaccination Mobile Program
Summer 2015

- Traveled with mobile team to outlying areas
- Administered vaccinations

Big Brother Volunteer 2015–present

Employment History
St. Mary's Medical Center: Williamsburg. Nursing assistant on cardiac unit.
2014–present

Ben's Bistro: Williamsburg. Lead waiter in a popular, busy urban restaurant
2010–2014

Honors and Professional Affiliations
Achieved perfect clinical attendance record

Member, American Nurses Association

Dean's list 2015, 2016, 2017

Chair Student Nurses Association 2017

Outstanding Scholar Award 2017

Recipient Nightingale Nursing Scholarship 2017

Learn more about résumés and cover letters at nursecode.com.

9

Cover Letters

*Everything you've ever wanted is on
the other side of fear.*

—*GEORGE ADDAI*

Have you ever felt that applying online is imper-sonal? That if only they could meet you in person, they would be wowed by your personality?

Well, a cover letter is the next best thing to meeting with a real person—a real person just like you, who enjoys a personal touch and a story. A cover letter or essay can be your golden ticket to getting noticed. Your cover letter should reflect your personality and energy. Include examples to make it authentic and memorable.

Do not recap your résumé in your cover letter. While cover letters and résumés have the same ultimate purpose—to *land an interview*—your résumé lists your work history and provides a summary of your skills, abilities, and accomplishments, tailored to the job you are seeking.

The purpose of a cover letter is to introduce yourself to the organization, pique their interest, compel them to read your résumé, and motivate them to interview you..

Both should highlight your skills relevant to the job you are applying for, and both should show that you are the best fit for the job.

When filling out an online application, you may be instructed to upload your cover letter. If there are no such instructions, look for a question such as "What haven't we asked about your skills, knowledge, or experience that you think is important to share?" That's your cue to include information about your background, skills, or work history that makes you uniquely qualified for the position and helps you to stand out from other applicants.

Finally, consider the tone. Mirror the culture. Hospitals are typically conservative organizations, so be conservative but not stiff or overly formal. Strike a professional but friendly and engaging tone that is authentic and true to you.

COVER LETTER BASICS

Limit your cover letter to one page, with three to five or six short paragraphs, in a pleasing layout with ample white space. White space provides contrast to dense text and gives your reader bite-size information a little at a time with a visual and mental break in between. Readers are more likely to leave their eyes on a document that provides visual respite.

You should not use artsy fonts or wild graphics unless you are applying to an artsy kind of industry (not nursing). When it comes to using multiple fonts, don't. Less is more. Times New Roman, Calibri, and Arial at a ten to twelve point size are clear and easy to read.

Make sure to include keywords from the job description in your online application. Application-tracking software (ATS) is programmed to pick up the keywords, skills, and experience for the job. If "leadership qualities" is listed in the job posting, use "leadership" or attributes of leadership in your cover letter.

Here's a great example from a large children's hospital that does a good job of describing what a good fit is in its job posting for RNs:

- Someone with an insatiable curiosity and sense of inquiry to learn why we treat cancer as we do—and to help us achieve the next level of care
- A heartfelt commitment to providing quality, evidence-based care to help patients achieve optimal outcomes
- An abiding compassion for patients and their families, all of whom are fighting against cancer and for a return to health
- A holistic view of healthcare, recognizing that professional nurses not only care for the physical symptoms of cancer but for the mental, emotional, psychological, and spiritual manifestations as well
- A genuine desire to be challenged by a complex patient population that is aging and may be suffering from comorbidities like heart disease or diabetes in addition to a cancer diagnosis
- A contagious enthusiasm for focusing—or refocusing—your career on the sense of vocation that compelled you to choose nursing in the first place

You can see that they are looking for nurses with a lot of heart, a spirit of clinical inquiry, and for those who share their values of holistic, patient-centered care. They have told you exactly what they are looking for in an employee. You should speak to those characteristics in your cover letter in a genuine, meaningful manner.

Avoid dull clichés, copycat buzzwords, and over-used terms because everyone uses them, they do not help you to stand out, and they don't say anything. The reader will tune out. Instead of saying *"detail-oriented, team-playing, results-producing, ethical"* give examples that illustrate the *detail-oriented, team-playing, results-producing, ethical* kind of awesome employee you are. As a bonus, you will have also demonstrated that you have excellent communication skills.

Instead of saying, "I'm a natural leader," say, "I led a community vaccination drive for our senior class project," or "I'm always picked as jury foreman and committee chair. I enjoy the responsibility and leading others." Personal examples are memorable and help you to stand out.

- Team player (try instead "I'm always picked to be on a team")

- Results driven (try instead "I set goals for my patient to achieve by the end of shift every day, such as increasing mobility")
- Strong work ethic (try instead "I had a perfect attendance record at my last job, and I take pride in being punctual")
- Detail oriented (now it's your turn to try)

OPENING

Your cover letter should reference the advertisement, job ID, and job title. Introduce yourself.

Do not use "To whom it may concern." Even though it may take some digging, find out the hiring manager's name to personalize the letter. You can call the hospital and ask who the manager of the nursing unit is, or call the floor and ask. The opening is where you mention if you're connected on LinkedIn, met at a job fair, or know someone in the organization.

MIDDLE

This is the strength part where you show them that you're a good fit; explain what you can do for their company (not why the job is good for you).

Never reference salary or make any work-related requests such as "my brother's wedding is in May."

Customize this section to your prospective employer. Before composing your new grad RN cover letter, research the organization. Be familiar with their mission statement, service lines, and culture. Are they for profit, not for profit, faith based? Do they do a lot of community work? Are they accredited in chest pain, stroke, and diabetes? Do they have a high turnover?

Describe how your skills and experience are a good fit for the organization, and why you're the right person for the job. It's about them, not you. Be their solution.

CLOSING

End your cover letter with a brief concluding paragraph. Reiterate your interest in the job. Summarize why you're a good fit.

Close with an *active call to action* and discuss the next steps. This could be "I will contact you early next week," "I look forward to setting a time to meet with you," or "I welcome the chance to speak with you." Avoid weak or overly passive endings such as "If interested, I hope you will contact me."

If you plan to follow up in one to two weeks, you can mention a specific date. If you prefer to leave the ball in their court, say that you look forward to discussing your qualifications further (but word it confidently to indicate that it's a given).

You might close by asking for a phone or Skype interview or an in-person interview. Whatever it is, it should move the process forward.

Again, check to see you've used the correct employer name, address, contact person, and contact person's title. Make sure you've used the correct date and have spelled the facility's name correctly. Don't forget to thank them for their time, perhaps offering some well wishes and good sentiments.

BUSINESS PRINT COPY FORMAT

The formatting in the sample letter I provide is a slight variation of a business type, with the recipient's contact information at the top, left centered. This is appropriate for a print copy. Leave four spaces between your closing ("sincerely," "best," and so on) for your typed name and your written signature.

E-MAIL FORMAT

If you are e-mailing your cover letter, leave out the recipient's contact information. Use the same salutation as in a business format.

Include the job you are applying for in the subject line of the e-mail. The e-mail subject line is very important. Here's an example: "RN New Grad Residency Position Application: Nicole Nurse."

The most important thing is to follow the employer's instructions precisely:

- Send cover letter as an e-mail attachment (if not specified, pdf or .docx).
- Send cover letter in body of e-mail (copy and paste it in).
- Send cover letter via e-mail and attach résumé (if not specified, pdf or .docx).

Your contact information should be at the bottom of the e-mail. Of course you will provide a professional e-mail address that is some combination of your first and last names (meaning don't use hotstuff@yahoo.com). Make sure your contact information is current, professional, and correct.

WAIT TO HIT SEND

- Set your cover letter aside for at least twenty-four hours without looking at it. Some typos have a habit of not showing up before then.

- In the meantime, have several friends with editing abilities review your cover letter. It must be free of mistakes.
- Review your cover letter for errors that the spell checker doesn't pick up. For example, you may have typed "form" instead of "from."
- A great way to review grammar and syntax is to read your cover letter word for word out loud.

Tip: Check for congruence. Make sure your cover letter information matches the information you provided in your résumé or job application. There should be no contradictions between the two.

CREATIVE STRATEGIES FOR COVER LETTERS

It's crucial that you capture the reader's interest instantly because it's estimated that you only have about six to ten seconds to do so. Here are a couple of optional tips guaranteed to capture their interest.

Add a PS: PS adds another unique touch. People's eyes are drawn to a PS. Sometimes it's read before the body of the letter! The one in the example below contains contact information.

Be creative, bold, and risky: Consider a banner headline at the top of your cover letter. It could say "Call me!" in large font. You will most assuredly stand out as it's pretty much guaranteed that no other applicants will use a headline.

This is risky because humor depends on the receiver's response, but it will be noticed. While not for everyone, it depends on your comfort level with risk.

> You get in life what you have the courage to ask for.
>
> —OPRAH WINFREY

Nicole Nurse

3000 Winning Way, Anytown, CO 95678
Cell: 555-777-1212 *nicole.nurse@gmail.com*
Linkedin.com/in/Nicole nurse

February 22, 2015 *(Use business letter format.)*

Diane Woods
Hiring Manager
2430 Prosperity Way
Anytown, CO 95678

Let me show you why I'm a perfect fit for your position! (Creative option.)

Dear Ms. Woods, *(Avoid "To whom it may concern.")*

I'm highly interested in the new grad RN opening in oncology at Happy Hospital. I will be graduating in May 2018 and taking the NCLEX on June 2, 2018. The values of compassion and dignity in your mission statement and dedication to community outreach resonate with me. *(Individualize to targeted employer.)*

I am especially interested in Happy Hospital because of your expanding oncology program. My grandmother had cancer, and helping my mother care for her as a teenager made me decide to become a nurse. My grandma died with dignity. I have compassion for patients and families who are dealing with illness and understand how difficult it is. (*Personalize by example. Stories are remembered.*)

My recent clinical rotations on 3 South at Happy Hospital gave me experience with a diverse patient population and a respect for cultural differences. The emphasis on patient satisfaction impressed me. I was pleased that my preceptor, June S., RN, and my clinical instructor, Sandra H., RN, both gave me high evaluations on my communication skills with patients and coworkers. It's due to practicing the skills I learned while taking the module "How to Deal with Patient Complaints." (*Highlight your strengths. Patient satisfaction is of high concern to all hospitals.*)

In addition to my nursing skills, I've developed strong leadership skills. As president of the Denver Chapter of the National Student Nurses' Association, I led a team that initiated a very successful Adopt a Family community program at Christmastime. The program was featured in the *Denver Times* and will be carried on by future nursing classes. (*Give concrete examples of skills rather than saying, "I'm a strong leader."*)

A letter and résumé can only tell you so much, and I would appreciate the opportunity to meet with you in person. I will contact you within a few days to discuss the next step. I look forward to meeting you, and please do not hesitate to contact me at 444-777-1212. (*Call to action in final paragraph—discuss next step—rather than a passive ending such as "I hope to hear from you."*)

Sincerely,
Nicole Nurse

Enclosure (1) résumé (*or attachment*)

PS—If you would like to meet with me sooner, you may reach me immediately on my cell at 444-777-1212. Thank you kindly for your time and consideration, Ms. Woods.

There is no need to add "references on request." The employer will ask for them at a later date.

CHAPTER SUMMARY AND CHECKLIST

- Is it spell checked?
- Does it include professional contact information?

- Did you close with an actionable call to action?

Visit nursecode.com for more examples of résumés and cover letters.

10

Essay Questions

Why sometimes I've believed as many as six impossible things before breakfast.

—*The Red Queen, Alice in Wonderland*

For some reason, and to your favor, nursing employers like to ask essay questions of nursing applicants, especially for entry to nursing residencies. For them, it's a method of narrowing down the hundreds of applications. For you, it's a way to stand out and shine. Think of it as nothing short of a golden opportunity.

It's very similar to writing an essay for a scholarship or for entry to nursing school. Give yourself plenty of time to compose your essay and enlist a family member or friend who is good at writing if needed. The employer will tell you how long it should be. Follow the same rules for layout and visual appeal.

What kinds of questions are asked? Here are some questions taken recently straight from the websites of several major hospitals.

- Why you are interested in our hospital?
- Describe a personal sacred encounter that you experienced during your nursing clinical rotation (question from a faith-based organization).
- Explain why you chose nursing as a major/ career.
- Why are you interested in our community, and what would you contribute as a nursing professional to our organization?
- What plans do you have for continued formal education/what are your goals for professional growth?

Application essays have a critical effect on your chances of landing an interview, a job, or a placement in nursing school. The challenge for you is make yours memorable. You can do that by using these five tips.

HOW TO WRITE A NURSING APPLICATION ESSAY

When asked to submit an essay along with your application for employment, the employer is using the essay as a way to screen applicants. All things being equal, the essay will help the employer to narrow down the list of candidates and can make the difference between landing an interview or not.

Many candidates will submit an uninteresting, cliché-ridden essay with grammatical errors. By contrast, if you follow these tips, your essay will stand out.

FOLLOW INSTRUCTIONS

It is highly important that you understand and follow instructions. You are being evaluated on your ability to do so. If the length is not specified, use no more than two pages.

The essay can take several forms. You may be asked to write a one-page essay on a single topic or question. Alternatively, you may be asked to pick from several questions such as:

- What made you decide to be a nurse?
- Why do you want to be a nurse here at St. John's?

ALLOW AMPLE TIME

You will probably find it more difficult to write about yourself than you anticipate. Do not put it off until the last minute. If writing is not your forte, allow yourself even more time to produce a professional product.

Your essay must be highly polished, and that takes drafting, editing, and rework. Any less and it will not be your best effort and will not be as effective as it should. When you are finished, put it down for at least twenty-four hours and then pick it up. You will find room for improvement. Have three other people proofread it.

BE THE RECRUITER

Put yourself in the recruiter's chair. Think how many times by eleven in the morning the recruiter has read, "I'm a people person" or "I want to help people." Now picture the recruiter picking up your essay and yet again reading, "I'm a people person" and "I want to help people." It's important to keep the recruiter's perspective in mind the entire time and with every sentence you compose.

Avoid broad generalizations, clichés, and platitudes. Be genuine and personal. Avoid being stiff and overly intellectual. Everyone responds to authenticity. This comes from connecting and through telling stories. Use a meaningful quote for interest and short paragraphs with enough white space to avoid dense blocks of text.

Stand out with stories. It's essential that you stand out from all the other applicants. Use details and personal examples to stand out and make yourself memorable.

Describe yourself in a way that illustrates your skills:

"I learned in clinical rotations to look past a patient's angry behavior and try to find out the why. One day, my patient was very angry that his discharge was delayed because the physician had not rounded. He was rude to me, but I just said, 'You seem very upset. Do you want to talk about it?' and he shared that his wife with Alzheimer's had been home alone for forty-eight hours, and he was worried about her. I was able to get the discharge order and send him home."

It's an engaging story that shows your people skills and compassion. Likewise:

"I always try to plan ahead so I'll be prepared. My patient had a low H&H, but before I called the

*doctor, I checked to see if he had any blood avail-
able or a type and cross. I also checked the chart
to see if he had religious objections to receiving
blood. It turns out he was a Jehovah's Witness, and
I was able to let the physician know."*

This illustrates critical thinking skills, and every nurse
manager is concerned with critical thinking.

BE A GOOD FIT

To speak to the question, "Why do you want to
work here?" you have to know something about and
understand the organization. When the recruiter
reads your essay, you want him or her to respond
with, "He or she would be a great fit. Let's get this
person on the phone now."

Study their website. Perhaps they are featuring a
service line they are proud of such as oncology services, stroke, or chest-pain center. Maybe they were
voted People's Choice by their community or have
badges on their site for awards. If they have been
distinguished by Healthgrades or Leapfrog, it will
be displayed on their site. Incorporate this knowledge into your essay.

In some way communicate that you are aware of
what they stand for in the community. Then go on to

explain how your skills and values align with theirs. For example, consider a hospital that bills itself as doing "sacred work" and is a Christian organization. Reflect if or how your values align with theirs, and speak to that. You will be seen as a good fit.

Highlight why you are an exceptional candidate— because you really are. Believe it.

11

Confidence: How to Have It

Never bend your head. Always hold it high. Look the world straight in the eye.

—HELEN KELLER

The following chapter is a post written for my blog, nursecode.com.

Maybe you have an upcoming interview. Congratulations! Or perhaps you're just looking ahead toward future interviews. Either way, thanks for coming here, and I believe that I can help you wherever you are in your journey. I've personally hired a countless number of nurses and learned a lot about job interviewing that I want to share with you.

What's the best thing about an interview? You can wow them with your presence. You *must* wow them with your presence. Here's how to bring your A game to the face-to-face interview and blow the competition away.

Confidence, Confidence, Confidence

I asked my good friend Jamie, director of our hospital's versant residency program, "Jamie, all things being equal, how does the hiring panel (consisting of managers, directors, and staff RNs) select the winning candidate?" Jamie reflected and said, "Confidence."

All things being equal, the *confident candidate gets the job*. "Gee, thanks, but that's no help," you may say. "Me? I'm not confident. I'm Nervous Nellie!"

You may not *feel* confident, but you can *appear* confident, which *makes* you confident. Here's how.

WOW THEM WITH CONFIDENCE

A confident interviewing presence can't be measured, but it's something that is recognized and can be learned.

Your confidence is assessed within seconds of you entering the room. Your confident interviewing presence makes you immediately likable and irre-sistible. Employers hire the candidates they like. The most qualified person in the world is not going to ge the job if he or she comes across as aloof or dull.

Interview presence is learned.

Before entering the room, stop. Focus. Breathe in. Breathe out. Summon up your positive energy. Picture yourself about to step onto a stage to receive an award, and your adoring audience awaits you.

STEP ONTO YOUR STAGE

Now enter the room. Have a big, warm, genuine smile. Do not be timid in your bearing or your walk. Project high energy because nursing takes ener-getic, fast-thinking, and fast-moving people. Don't convey slowness or hesitation.

Immediately approach the interviewer(s) and extend your hand. Give a firm handshake. It takes a lot to compensate for a limp handshake.

When answering questions, do not look away, up, or down. Lean forward slightly and maintain eye con-tact with the questioner. While speaking, go around the table and make eye contact with each person.

Don't skip anyone. When you first catch their eyes, widen your eyes slightly. (Women know how to do this; it's subliminal flirting, but it's not taken as such. It's taken as interest.)

CONFIDENT POSTURE

Did you know that good posture alone increases self-esteem and confidence? There's a reason our mothers told us to "Sit up straight!" Do not allow your back to touch the back of the chair when seated. Keep your shoulders back and relaxed.

Excellent bearing, carriage, and posture assure that you will stand out by default. People assume you are successful and confident when you carry yourself well.

STRANGE CONFIDENCE-BUILDING EXERCISE

This may sound strange, but try it at home. Stand up. Take a big breath in. Strike a body-building pose.

The Hulk has confidence!

Picture the Hulk. Do the Hulk pose. Be the Hulk. Be big. Bigger! Watch out that your shirt doesn't rip open! Note how you feel. Shy? No! Powerful? Yes! (Men probably know this one.)

Note: I am not saying to walk into your interview like the Hulk. I am saying to become familiar with that bodily feeling of power and confidence and to practice summoning it up at will.

Did you know that Matthew McConaughey thumps his chest before starting a scene to loosen up and not be nervous?

CONFIDENT, PROFESSIONAL APPEARANCE

Ladies, consider getting your hair done the day of your interview. If you don't need a cut, have it blown out and styled. You will look polished and feel more confident. Men, be well groomed. Be familiar with the dress norms in your area.

Dress conservatively. Dressing conservatively shows respect by sublimating your individual dress style to that of the organization's image.

> *Please tell millennials not to show up for their interviews in the casual yoga pants, tank tops, and flip-flops style of dressing. And remind them to leave their cell phones in the car or turn them off.*
>
> —*From a recruiter*

Invest in a classy, classic outfit that you can wear for years to come, not a trendy one. Tempted to show the world your artsy, colorful, cutting-edge self? Great—but not in a nursing interview. Know the organization's policy on tattoos and piercings, and dress accordingly.

Your clothes should fit, flatter, and be functional. Functional means that if your pencil skirt does not have a kick pleat in the back, you will walk with minced steps and your skirt will ride up your thighs when you sit. Skip the perfume and colognes.

MANAGE YOUR NERVOUSNESS

You already know if you're a fast talker. I am. The solution is to practice strategies to lessen your nervousness because the real problem is nerves. Record yourself on your phone and practice slowing it down. It will sound uncomfortably slow but only to you.

If you think you talk too much, you probably do. Answer the questions but don't ramble tangentially. If you find yourself talking about your family or pets, you've gone on too long. Notice the body language of the interviewers. You can tell when you've lost interest.

Warning: If the interviewer is all chatty and casual, respond in kind, but remain professional. They are not your chummy friend; they are your interviewers, and they are assessing you.

CONFIDENCE SPECIFIC TO THE JOB REQUIREMENTS

Deep down, *you* have to believe that you are the best candidate for the job. Once you believe this, you will find your voice and be able to articulate as much to the interviewer.

If you have not identified your marketable assets, do this.

- Assess your personality, traits, and character-meaning make a list. Enlist the help of a couple of people who know you well because you need an outside perspective. Also, if you hear the same trait mentioned more than once from different sources, you'll internalize it and believe it. Add what they say to your list.
- Carry the list around, pull it out frequently, and look at it. This is your fabulous list, the list of you. It may include traits such as being passionate, caring, determined, dedicated, detailed, loyal, creative, analytical, and a team player (I would love to hear what your list says).
- Now look at the list of job requirements for the job you want. Hmm! You may see that

they are looking for someone who is detail oriented and compassionate with strong teamwork and problem-solving skills.

- Finally, cross match the lists to see what a great fit you are for them.

Be courteous to everyone from the minute you step onto the campus. It's the right thing to do, and for all you know, Kaitlin, the front desk person, may be the ICU nurse manager's niece.

Be authentic. The best you is the authentic you. Everyone responds to realness and genuineness. Confidence is half the key, and you are already a winner! Look how far you've come and imagine how far you'll go!

> Today you are you! That is truer than true! There is no one alive who is you-er than you!
>
> You have brains in your head. You have feet in your shoes. You can steer yourself any direction you choose.
>
> —Dr. Seuss

12

Interviews: General

Believe and act as if it were impossible to fail.

—C*HARLES* K*ETTERING*

You really, really want the job. You just know you'd be perfect for the position if only they'd give you a chance. But first comes the interview.

The only place Jonathan had ever wanted to work was the emergency department (ED) at Happening Hospital. Jonathan knew he would make a great ED nurse. He applied six long weeks ago and had almost given up. Competition was tough for the two open positions. But then his phone vibrated.

"Hello. May I speak to Jonathan Ward, please?"

"Yes. Yes, this is Jonathan."

"We're interviewing candidates for the ED on Thursday. We would like for you to come in at two o'clock. Will that work for you?"

"Yes. Yes! I mean yes, thank you. Yes, I'll be there."

When applicants are landing multiple interviews but not landing job offers, the culprit is their interview skills. In this chapter, you will learn how to positively stand out in your interview.

BE THE MEMORABLE ONE

Be memorable at every opportunity. For example, wear a memorable piece of jewelry such as a flower or a bird pin or perhaps a timepiece pinned to your shirt or jacket. Why? At the end of a long day of interviewing, the panel interviewers will find it hard to remember who said what even when they take notes. But if someone says, "The one with the peacock pin," you will be instantly recalled to memory.

Here's a typical conversation among interviewers at the end of day:

"Which one was it that went to UCSF—the one with the big glasses?"

"No, no, that was Ashley; she came in right before lunch, or maybe it was midmorning. She's the one with a sick brother, right? Or was that Angela?"

"No, Ashley was the one with the peacock pin, remember?"

"Oh, that's right! Ashley...she was very well pre-pared, don't you think? Let's pull her answers and résumé again."

Caution: Overall, your appearance should be well groomed and conservative. This is not the time to show your individualistic, artsy self. Cover any tattoos since many organizations require their employees to do so. Tattoos are much more likely to work against you than for you in the conservative healthcare industry, so it is prudent to cover them. Later on as an employee, you will be informed of the dress code as far as tattoos and piercings.

There must be zero clothing malfunctions. For women, check your button-down shirt for *gaposis*. Plan ahead. Do not put an outfit together for the first time on the day of your interview. Avoid any distracting apparel or anything remotely suggestive.

The focus should be on you, not on your body, your clothing, or your makeup.

Avoid wearing scrubs if at all possible. When you wear scrubs, you forfeit the opportunity to present yourself as a well-dressed, savvy candidate who understands business attire. Make every effort to schedule your interview on a day when you are not working in order to dress accordingly and give the interview your undivided attention.

EXUDE CONFIDENCE

Don't forget the most important thing to bring to your interview: confidence. I recently asked Lynda, the Director of Recruiting at our hospital, "What's the main thing you look for in a candidate?" Without missing a beat, she replied, "Positive self-esteem."

You don't have to feel 100 percent confident in order to portray confidence. Portraying confidence is a function of body posture, being articulate, and being prepared. Remember that *they picked you*; they already like you. Here's a secret: We (interviewers and managers) want you to succeed. Members on the interview panel are pulling for you. You can do this.

- Handshake: Your handshake works for or against you. It should be firm, not limp. At the same time, you should be making eye contact.

- Power posing: Try power posing in the bathroom just before your interview.
- Anxiety: Control your anxiety. Anxiety is often linked to perfectionism and can cause you to freeze. Let it go and be yourself. Practice relaxing techniques beforehand.
- Physical location rehearsal: Do a dry-run rehearsal. Prior to your interview, drive to the designated location at the same time of day as your interview. Park your car and go inside to find the interview location.
- Be courteous to all assistants you encounter because it's the right thing to do and because the front desk assistant may be the hiring manager's cousin.
- Consider getting your hair blown out and styled on the day of your interview to increase your confidence in your appearance.

- Never be late. Be ten to fifteen minutes early.
- Never carry a drink in hand. It makes you look too casual, and you might spill it.
- Never handle your phone. Mute it and put it away.
- Never be unprepared. Know as much about the company as you possibly can.

- Never forget copies of your résumé, license, CPR card, and the like. Bring extra copies.
- Never bring up the topic of salary or benefits. That comes later.

FIRST IMPRESSIONS

From the moment you enter the room, you are under scrutiny. Be prepared to make a good first impression. There are no second chances to make a first impression. Introverts and low-energy people must dig deep within themselves to muster up some social energy and sparkle for the duration of the interview.

The first ninety seconds are critical. Instant judgments are made about you in that time, including, "Will she or he fit in here?" Positive presence can be learned. It's how others read your personal energy, vibe, or aura, whatever you want to call it. First impressions are a function of facial expression, body language, bearing, appearance, and confidence. Your body is telling others all about you before your voice speaks. It's more than what you say; it's how you say it.

In two recent interviews, my inner voice said, "Hire this person" *before they even sat down.* I have talked with other interviewers who've experienced the same instant conviction.

Shake hands (space permitting) and make eye contact with each panel interviewer. Candidates who project warmth the instant they walk in the room score bonus points. After all, they are going to be working with patients. Project openness and warmth. Be humble but confident. Visualize yourself getting the job as a mental warm-up activity, but without being cocky.

Be open and authentic. Being overly guarded poses a risk-averse situation for the manager. If a manager can't read you because your face is immobile and your voice is monotone, he or she will not be willing to take a chance on you.

Managers look for openness, teachability, and a willingness to learn.

Be calm. Pregame nerves are natural, but remember that they already like you. They picked you. You're here because you have the right qualifications and potential.

WHAT TO BRING TO YOUR NURSING INTERVIEW

Jonathan has already:

- Planned what he will wear.

- Planned where to park and knows where the interviewing space is.
- Practiced his interview questions.

PORTFOLIO

Now all that's left is to prepare his portfolio. But wait, what *is* a portfolio anyway? And how can a new grad have one? The better question is: what do you bring to a nursing interview? There are no hard and fast rules, but here are some helpful guidelines.

First of all, bring whatever they ask you to bring, if anything. This shows you can and do follow instructions. This could be a copy of your license or anything else.

Bring a copy of your résumé on heavyweight, quality paper. Often the interviewing panel will have been provided résumés, but it doesn't hurt. It shows a prepared, professional applicant. Even though a résumé handed out during an interview may not count *for* you, it can still count *against* you. I have seen résumés with glaring typos.

Bring a copy of your nursing license, BLS, ACLS, and any other certifications copied onto a sheet of paper. BLS and ACLS cards look best printed in color. Be sure to align the cards neatly on the printer so that the print copy looks nice.

Bring letters of reference on quality paper. Letters of reference may not be read at the time of the interview but may be referred to later when tiebreaker discussions are taking place.

Bring enough packets—and then extras. If the recruiter tells you that it is going to be a panel interview with five interviewers, bring ten copies. There is nothing to prevent the nurse manager from grabbing another nurse or two on the way to the interview and saying, "Come with me." It's awkward and dissatisfying for one person on the interview panel not to have a packet when those to the left and right do.

Worried about walking in with an armload of folders? Use a laptop carrying bag or satchel. Both look smart with any outfit, are gender neutral, and are functional.

Bring a notepad and pen for your own use to takes notes. Taking a brief note at the right time implies deference and attention.

It's not necessary to include transcripts. They can be lengthy and are basically uninteresting. It's a given that you attended clinical rotations and took required classes. A GPA over 3.75 sets you apart but can be included in your résumé.

Place your documents in a simple paper file folder or two-pocket file folder. Confidently hand a port-folio packet to each interviewer. Make eye contact and smile. They'll notice your awesomeness.

The best portfolio packet I've ever seen was Amanda's. She brought dark-blue paper folders with a business card affixed to the front bottom cor-ner. Her business card included a picture of herself, contact information, and a favorite quote. (Never put your photo on a résumé.) What made including a business card with an image such a good idea? After a long day of interviewing candidate after candidate, it's easy for even the most conscien-tious, note-taking interviewer to mix up candidates and details. At the after-interview discussions, my eyes kept being drawn to her smiling business card image, and it was easy to recall how she answered her questions.

IF YOU FREEZE DURING AN INTERVIEW

This is taken from my blog, nursecode.com.

You're interviewing, and the interviewers ask you a question that you are not prepared for. Let's say they ask, "Tell us about a time you overcame an obstacle at work." You go completely blank. You try to access your brain, but there's only an empty space where your brain used to be—a void.

Your eyes widen, your mouth opens, but no words come out. Six sets of eyes stare at you expectantly, and you have—nothing. It's not pretty when it happens, and you have to be able to move quickly into recovery and damage control. Here's what to do.

Acknowledge

Own it. Apologize. Smile and say, *"I'm sorry. I'm having a brain freeze."* Sharing your embarrassment wins favor and breaks tension. Everyone has had such a moment. The interviewers will put themselves in your shoes and empathize. They are now squarely on your side.

Ask for a favor

People like to grant favors. Smile and ask, *"Can we move on or circle back later to this question? I seem to be drawing a serious blank on this one."* By asking for a favor, you have now allowed them to be gracious and generous.

Use humor

Humor is a two-edged sword to be used carefully and with finesse. When skillfully used, it's a powerful tool. To use it successfully, you have to:

- Read the vibe in the room.
- Have great timing. Hesitation ruins an otherwise clever remark.
- Deliver your line with confidence and without hesitation.

Self-effacing humor is usually the most effective: *"Oh, no! My mother told me this might happen. I hate when she's right,"* or *"I think I need a brain reboot."*

Deflect

Say, for example, that the employer asked, "Tell us about a time you disagreed with a supervisor and how you handled it." You blank. Smile and say, "I am temporarily drawing a blank on that one. Can I tell about you a time when I…" Then proceed with a prepared example that highlights one of your skills—maybe conflict management, teamwork, ethics, or patient/customer satisfaction.

Move on

Don't shame yourself, and don't stay in that place. Do not let this define your interview. Smile widely. It is a natural human reaction to freeze when you are taken by surprise or are in danger (freeze, fight, or flee). The interviewers know this.

Some of the best nurses and quick thinkers in patient situations don't have the quick-thinking interview skill. It is not an indicator of being an excellent nurse. So if that's you, it's OK but you want to be prepared by having your move-on backup plan ready.

What I've seen

One young woman froze but wasn't able to recover. She did everything but cry. It was clear she was devastated and couldn't move forward in the interview. All the interviewers were understanding, but feeling bad for a candidate does not mean they'll hire that candidate. Jason, one of the interviewers, said kindly, "It's OK. Take a moment. Shake it off," but she wasn't able to.

By contrast, another candidate blanked, shook his head, and smiled ruefully. "I should have this, but I don't." We all laughed in relief that he broke the tension. He shifted in his chair and asked, "Would you mind if we come back to this or move on to the next question? I need some more time." He moved past the moment smoothly and impressed us with his poise.

The first interviewer made us all feel uncomfortable for a prolonged amount of time. The second interviewer won us over and made us laugh.

PREPARATION IS THE BEST PREVENTION

Being prepared lessens your chances of being blindsided in an interview.

Do what you think you cannot do. You can, you know!

13

Video Interviews

Believe you can and you're halfway there.

—*THEODORE ROOSEVELT*

Video interviews may be conducted as a first-round interview or as a hiring interview for long-distance candidates.

SET THE STAGE FOR YOUR VIDEO INTERVIEW

Pick a space with a neutral background. The focus should be you and not a distracting wall hanging.

Inspect the room carefully. A friend of mine chose her bedroom for her video interview. Everything seemed fine until the interview ended, and she turned around and spotted a lacy bra tossed over the back of a chair in full view of the camera.

Close the door and keep your pets out. Dogs and cats will uncannily know the recording area is out of bounds and therefore stalk you accordingly during your interview.

Silence all phones and alarms in the vicinity. Put a notice on the front door saying not to ring the doorbell.

LIGHTS, CAMERA, ACTION

Lighting is critical to your video nursing interview. Bright, natural lighting is best with lighting both in front of and behind you.

If you wear glasses, make sure the light is not shining in your eyes (coming toward you) and reflecting off your lenses. Make sure your face is not in shadow. Rehearse the lighting setup ahead of time at the time of day you will be interviewing.

Position your webcam so you are neither looking up nor down at the interviewer. Check the lens of your camera to make sure it's clean.

DRESS FOR SUCCESS

Dress as you would for a live interview and not just from the waist up. It's important to mentally be in full interview mode, which is hard if you are wearing a nice business shirt but are barefoot with cutoff jean shorts underneath.

Avoid wearing all white as you will appear washed out. Do not wear clothing the same color as the background, or you will fade into the background. The color red does not translate well. Avoid busy prints as they are distracting. Women can wear more makeup than usual as it translates well on camera.

ACT THE PART

Less than 10 percent of your communication is through words. The majority is your facial expression, tone of voice, and body language. The second you are live on camera, the interviewer is forming an impression of you and mostly through your appearance.

Project warmth and energy. Sit up straight. Be *on*. Smile appropriately and listen attentively. Resist looking at yourself on the screen; instead, make eye contact with your interviewer by looking directly at the webcam. Lean in slightly to show interest and engagement.

TECHNICALITIES

Be sure you have enough battery life on your device. Choose a location where your Internet connection is reliable. Be flexible and gracious if technical problems arise. If there are video problems, the interview can always be conducted as a phone interview.

NOT LIVE

A video nursing interview is not the same as a face-to-face interview. There is a slight time lag. When asked a question, nod to give a second or two and to avoid talking over the interviewer.

Unlike in a live interview, you can have notes nearby or even posted on the wall behind the camera to remind you of what to say like a teleprompter.

PREPARE AND REHEARSE

Don't be lulled into not preparing because you are in a comfortable location such as your home. This is not casual FaceTime between friends; it is a job interview. Rehearse your answers, and be fully prepared.

You didn't come this far only to come this far, my friend.

14

Behavioral Interview Questions

What we fear doing most is usually what we most need to do.

—*Tim Ferriss*

Nursing interviews typically include behavioral questions that are designed to test for specific characteristics required/desired for your job. In this chapter, we'll cover some commonly asked behavioral interview questions.

They generally start with "Tell me about a time," "Give us an example," or "Describe a situation." They are designed to give the employer insight into how you would respond to similar situations in the future based on your past behavior.

The manner in which you answer the question is telling. It isn't about confessing your weaknesses, exposing yourself, and being overly vulnerable. It's about demonstrating confidence, honesty, and composure when presented with a behavioral interview question. Show some personality. Don't be timid. Remember that *stories are remembered*, so be prepared to tell some stories.

PREPARE THESE THREE EXAMPLES

To start with, prepare three to four examples. Examples make you memorable. Examples are short stories with a purpose, and stories are remembered.

To prepare your examples, anticipate characteristics the employer will be looking for. Their questions will be designed to test for those characteristics. For example, you could reasonably expect that an RN employer may want to know about your:

- **Personal ethics and insight**: "Tell us about a time when you made a critical mistake at work."
- **Customer service**: "Give us an example of a time when you went above and beyond in customer service."
- **Conflict management:** "Describe a conflict with a coworker and how you resolved it."

- **Flexibility:** "Tell me about a time you had to adjust to a change at work."

Now think back. Recall a concrete example of going above and beyond in customer service. Think of a time when you made a serious mistake, disagreed with a supervisor, faced an ethical dilemma, and so on. As you think back, more examples will come to mind.

Be sure to include at least one example of how you benefited a former employer through your customer service skills as patient satisfaction is high on hospital radars..

Your examples can come from school, work, or life experience because what they all have in common is you and your behavior—behavior that illustrates the characteristics they are looking for in a candidate.

When composing your examples, follow this helpful formula:

- Briefly describe the situation.
- Identify the challenges you encountered.
- Explain the action steps you took.
- Share the outcome.
- Summarize what you learned and how you will apply it moving forward.

Tip: Your prepared examples may not exactly match the question, but that's OK. For example, if you are asked, "Tell us about a time you observed a coworker doing something unethical and what you did about it," you can say, "I haven't really had that experience, but there *was* a time when I disagreed with a coworker." The interviewers will go with it.

REHEARSE

Interviews are not the time to wing it. Be prepared. When you're not prepared, you're liable to freeze, skip all over the place, or ramble and never stop talking. Rehearse your answers with a friend several times. You can also record yourself and play the recording back to critique yourself. The purpose is not to memorize—because you want to retain your spontaneity—but to recall your talking points. Each time you practice out loud will be a slightly different version while retaining the key message and content.

- Compose examples using the formula above.
- Rehearse and practice ahead of time with a friend.
- Practice again with someone else.
- Don't memorize your answer but commit your talking points to memory and get them in.

- Don't repeat and don't ramble; you will lose your punch.

Let's look at the most commonly asked behavioral interview questions.

TELL US ABOUT YOURSELF

Have you ever been on a date with someone new? If so, you've been asked this question. So you *already have experience* in choosing what to share about yourself. It's the same in an interview.

Decide what to share about yourself by including examples that highlight the traits and characteristics they are looking for in a candidate. Focus on what most interests the interviewer, and stress your accomplishments.

- Put yourself in their shoes. Practice and listen to yourself from their point of view.
- Talk in stories. Stories are remembered.
- Be relevant. It's probably not relevant to landing a nursing position in ICU that you moved from New York to Idaho when you were twelve, but it is relevant and memorable that you decided to become a nurse when your younger sibling was hospitalized.

Present-past-future model

One way to structure your answer to the "tell us about yourself" interview question is to use the present-past-future model.

- Tell them where you are now (present) in your job situation.
- Mention your previous work placement (past).
- Close with talking about your hope to be employed by them (future).

Here's an example of how to answer "tell me about yourself" using the present-past-future model:

Present

(Smiling): "Well, currently I'm in my last semester of nursing school. I'm class president and received the Florence Nightingale Award for exemplary patient care and academic standing. Before that and up until last summer, I worked as a nursing assistant."

Past

"For the three years that I was a CNA, I had perfect attendance and organized the monthly unit birthday parties. I always tend to get involved in whatever group I'm in. I'm very social, and I get my energy from interacting with people and working in teams. Last summer, I interned as a student nurse on med surg at Happy Hospital in the same town where I attend university. The nurse manager asked me to stay on and work as an RN on her floor. She said she really liked the way I interact with patients. It's probably because I learned a lot from a module I took called 'How to handle patient complaints."

Future
"But family is most important to me, and I miss my nieces and nephews. I grew up snowboarding in the winter and can't wait to go snowboarding again. Now that I'm moving back to my hometown, I'm really looking forward to an opportunity to work here at Happier Community Hospital, where I can begin my career as an RN and grow."

Here the applicant started in the present, segued to the past, and ended optimistically in the future. She or he also said (in code), "I am a leader, a people person, a self-starter, savvy (I understand about patient satisfaction), and loyal," right?

> Tip: Remember to smile. You look beautiful when you smile.

WHY SHOULD WE HIRE YOU?
"Why should we hire you?" is a classic interview question and one for which you must be prepared. It's your chance to show how you meet the employer's needs.

Variations of the interview question: "We have a lot of applicants. Why should we hire you over all the other candidates?"

What the employer is looking for: That you can articulate what makes you stand out, that you are confident, and that you understand that you are here to help them meet their challenges.

How to answer: This question is often posed at the end of the interview and may be your last chance to sell yourself to the interviewer. Reaffirm that you are a team player, and tell them why you are the best candidate for the position. Have three reasons (talking points) ready for your answer—"You should hire me because…"—and give them your three reasons.

Answer completely but be succinct. Master your delivery. Be confident, smile, and make eye contact with each person. Convince them that they should hire you before another employer snaps you up.

WHY SHOULD WE HIRE YOU? EXAMPLES

"My ability to work well with others and perform well under stress makes me a good match to work in your fast-paced emergency department. I've wanted to work here since last summer, when I heard several members of your ED got together and traveled up

to Lake Isabella to help volunteer in the fire. I have a volunteer heart as well, and it's just the kind of team I'd like to be a part of."

If you live out of area, you have an extra challenge. You have to reasonably convince the interviewers that you are not going to leave in two years and go back to a location more desirable. If you have family or a love interest in the area, it helps your case. Once on a panel interview, a candidate from out of town was asked, "Tell us why we should hire you. We have several applicants that live in the area."

She replied, "I can tell you are looking for nurses who will stay in the area. I've been looking to relocate, and my cousins have been trying to get me to move here. I would love to live in the same town as them and help take care of Grandma. I would be so excited to be able tell them I'm moving here. I tend to be very loyal, and once I settle in someplace, I stay. I'm looking for a work family where I can grow as an RN and find my niche."

Don't compare yourself to other candidates even if asked, "Why should we hire you over the other candidates?" Simply say, "I can't speak to the other candidates' abilities, but I can tell you about mine."

WHAT'S YOUR BEST STRENGTH?

Beforehand, do some self-reflection and identify your strengths. You have to know yourself before you can tell anyone else who you are. It helps to ask a couple of people who know you well, "What would you say are my best strengths?"

Next, look at what the employer is seeking: an RN who is competent with a good attitude and who is loyal. Finally, match the two—your strengths with the employer's needs. Tell them your strengths in story form or by giving examples. Stories are remembered.

- Are you a natural leader—always the group project leader, class president, and jury foreman?
- Are you caring? One applicant said she cared for her grandmother at home in her last days of a long illness and admired the hospice nurses. She knew then she was going to be a nurse. She also said she has been a caring, caretaker type of person all her life.
- Are you highly organized and efficient? Maybe you were a waitress and have mastered the skill set of juggling ten things at a time (prioritization). Or maybe you've organized a large wedding or your class graduation. Give examples. Speak in stories.

WHAT ARE YOUR BEST STRENGTHS? EXAMPLES:

"I'm told I'm really likable, and it's true; I get along with everyone. It's one of my main strengths; I've always been that way. I talk easily with strangers, and people always seem to open up and confide in me."

"All my life and all the way back to grade school, people have wanted me on their teams, whether it's sports or group projects. In nursing school, everyone wanted me to be in their study groups. I enjoy being on a team and working together to accomplish a common goal. I get my energy from connecting with others."

In the first example, the applicant is showing them what good social skills she or he has without saying, "My social skills are excellent, and I am trustworthy." In the second example, the applicant is saying that she or he is a team player and an extrovert.

Healthcare facilities prefer to hire people who work well with others, have good social skills, get along well with patients and visitors, and can pull together as a team for the sake of patient care.

Do not say, "I'm a hard worker." Instead, give an example. Now you give it a try and see how you could give an example of the hard worker you are without simply saying, "I'm a hard worker."

GIVE AN EXAMPLE OF A TIME...

The employer may ask "Give us an example of a time you went above and beyond in your patient care"

What the employer is looking for: Customer service is king right now as patient satisfaction scores are high on hospital radars. Demonstrate that you understand the importance of patient satisfaction in the industry. Show how you will help them achieve higher patient satisfaction scores.

Variations of the interview question: *"Tell us about a time you went out of your way to meet a customer's expectations." "Tell us when you advocated for a patient."*

How to answer: Tell a compelling story. Give an example of how you benefited a former employer through your customer service skills, or think of a time in clinical when you went over and above on behalf of a patient or family. Instead of saying, "I excel at customer service," give an example:

One day in clinical, I had a Spanish-speaking patient. He was nervous and waiting for his daughter. It was the end of our shift and time for the postclinical conference, but I just knew it wasn't a good time to leave him. I asked my instructor if it would be OK if I stayed over long enough to continue translating for him until his daughter arrived. I'm fluent in Spanish.

She said it would be all right, and I stayed at his bedside until his daughter came. It turned out he was embarrassed to ask for a urinal, and I was able to get one for him and provide privacy. I really like when I have a chance to help someone like that. I'm the one who feels blessed.

Practice your story until you know you won't leave out any key points, but never memorize it. You want to sound honest and authentic, not overrehearsed.

TELL US ABOUT A CONFLICT AT WORK

Variations of the interview question: "Describe a time when you disagreed with your boss." "Tell me about a difficult patient and how you handled the situation." "Describe a conflict with a coworker and how you resolved it."

What the employer is looking for: Conflict resolution skills, interpersonal skills, teamwork, and that you interact well with others. The focus should be on your ability to resolve conflict in a professional and positive manner.

How to answer: Ideally, have three examples ready, one of conflict with your boss, one with a coworker, and one with a customer/patient. Segue if needed ("While I haven't had *that* particular experience, I *have* had..."). Then give a similar example that shows your ability to communicate with others and come to a working agreement. They will go with it.

Briefly describe the situation. Speak to the action you took. Share the positive results. Here is an example:

> *I was working on a nursing unit as a PCT during school, and one other PCT, Edna, seemed to be giving me a hard time. For example, she would take my blood pressure machine without asking and "forget" to give it back.*
>
> *I was frustrated but also puzzled. I hadn't done anything to provoke her. I just stayed calm and tried to see things from her point of view and not take it personally. Then it dawned on me. Edna was the senior PCT on the floor, having been there for over fifteen years. I had just recently been hired to the unit and had*

been given a choice schedule due to being in school. The nurse manager paid me a lot of attention as she was recruiting me to work there as soon as I graduated.

The next shift Edna and I worked together, I went down to the Starbucks on campus and got a flat white coffee for myself and her. We can't drink beverages in the nursing station, so I said, "Hey, come on and take a break with me." I asked her about herself and discovered she is a single mom with three teenagers. She said she always wanted to be a nurse but couldn't afford to go to school with three kids to raise. After we talked for a bit, I said I needed to ask her a favor. I said, "Edna, I notice you really know how to get your post-op hip patients up out of bed to the chair. I've been afraid to move them because I'm not good at hip precautions. Can you teach me?" She smiled and said, "Sure."

It turned out that Edna taught me a lot I didn't know. I had been using the temporal thermometer wrong, and she showed me the right way. She taught me how to do a linen change with a bedbound patient like a pro. I noticed that my blood pressure *machine didn't disappear any longer, and Edna seemed to have lost her resentment of me. My grandma always told me to put yourself in the other person's shoes, and I guess she was right.*

WHAT'S YOUR GREATEST WEAKNESS?

Your stomach's churning just thinking about how to answer the "what's your greatest weakness?" nursing interview question. It is a nerve-wracking question, but it won't be, once you're prepared. In fact, it is a golden opportunity. Good news! By the end of this section, you'll be able to confidently answer this interview question as well as know the answers never to give.

What the employer is looking for: The first thing to understand is that they don't really want the truth. They definitely don't want to know your personal weaknesses (you binge on ice cream, you're insecure, you get jealous). You won't get points for candidly coming clean and telling them you forget your mother's birthday. It's designed to see if you demonstrate self-awareness and are willing to adapt. Then how should you answer this question?

How to answer: Strategically. Whenever you have to talk about a negative such as a weakness in an interview, skillfully guide it into a positive as soon as you can while still owning the weakness. When they think about you, you want them to have positive associations.

No more than a third of your words should be spent on describing your weakness. A brief, matter-of-fact statement is best. Don't repeat yourself, and don't go into unnecessary detail. Focus on your self-growth and development.

How to choose your weakness

Your goal is to present a genuine weakness that does not damage your potential for the position but also does not come across as unrealistic or staged. When choosing your weakness, pick something work related and fixable. Make sure that it's not something critical to the job but that it is something germane to the job.

- Frame your weakness as an opportunity you've identified for professional improvement and growth (*self-awareness*).
- Describe the progress you've made in a story or example (*positive*).

- Give an example of what action steps you've taken (*positive*).
- Don't dwell on the negative.
- End on a positive note.

What not to choose as your weakness
Don't say, "I'm no good with Excel" because this is not a skill set needed for a clinical bedside nurse. It will be seen as chickening out or skirting the question.

Don't say, "I struggle with math calculations" because you are going to be passing medications, and your aptitude and safety will be brought into question.

Avoid "I work too much," "I'm a workaholic," or "I'm a perfectionist" as these are overused, and they will know you Googled your answer. These responses show that you did not prepare for this question in a meaningful, authentic way.

YOUR GREATEST WEAKNESSES EXAMPLES

"I'm working on my time management skills. I'm learning to batch my duties whenever possible and to carry enough needed supplies with me. When I

anticipate what my patients might need, I'm better prepared and save time."

"English is my second language. I read and write well, but I want to be more comfortable with idiomatic English. I'm taking English as a second language course at the community college."

"I don't always delegate as much as I should because it's uncomfortable, and I always want to do everything myself. I've come to see that delegating is important in order to work as a team and get everything done. On every shift on my last rotation, I made it a point to delegate more each day. It's still out of my comfort zone, but I'm improving daily."

Note that none of the above examples used the word "weakness" when answering. The focus is on the positive.

Tip: Be prepared with two answers as you may be asked, "What are your greatest weaknesses (plural)?"

15

Situational Interview Questions

You're off to great places! Today is your day! Your mountain is waiting, so get on your way!

—Dr. Seuss

et's say you just landed an interview for your dream job in ICU. Or maybe you landed an interview for the ED. Congratulations! You have been selected from among numerous candidates, and now it's finally your chance to shine.

Ashley landed a new grad interview for tele and stayed up all night studying arrhythmia strips, concentrating on heart blocks. The next morning she was tired and frazzled. Driving to her interview, she kept thinking of clinical questions they might ask that she wasn't prepared for.

The temptation is to bone up on the specialty so they'll see how knowledgeable you are and hire you. That's not how it works. Relax. Don't brush up on your arrhythmia strips for tele or chemo drug antiemetics for oncology. Likewise, don't cram on the conduction system of the heart.

They know you're new. They know you're smart. And they know you don't have experience. They are fully prepared to train the candidate who is a good fit—as long as the candidate is competent and safe.

This is not to say you should not prepare. You are wise to prepare because the candidate who is prepared is more confident and interviews far better than the candidate who is unprepared. So definitely do prepare but not in the way you think. Here's what you will be asked, and here's how you need to answer.

PRINCIPLES OF SITUATIONAL QUESTIONS

The most important thing is to illustrate that you're a safe practitioner. Here are the responses they are looking for regardless of the scenario.

- Stay with the patient. *You must say this in so many words.*

- Call for help. *This is most important and shows that you recognize your own limitations as a new nurse.*
- Provide support and any on-the-spot interventions you can: *vital signs, oxygen, reposition, and so on.*

They are looking to see if you are safe and competent. It's really as simple as that.

THE BASIC CLINICAL SCENARIO

You will be presented with a clinical scenario. The details will vary according to the specialty area, but the story line will remain the same.

A picture will be painted of a patient who has a sudden change of condition and is now experiencing some kind of distress (fell, is clutching her chest in pain, is bleeding, became diaphoretic, is confused, and the like). Don't read too much into it. They are not trying to trick you.

Typically, you are the only person in the room when this sudden change of condition occurs. An interviewer turns to you and says, "What do you do?" Know that they are not expecting a diagnosis, nor are they testing to see if you recall the intricacies of the Kreb cycle. The interviewers are listening carefully to see if you are safe, to see if you understand your role, and to see if you exhibit critical thinking.

CLINICAL CUES

When you are given a patient scenario, the interviewers will give you clues to cue your answer. Listen for them. They will include key clinical descriptions such as "respiratory rate of twenty-four" and "SOB." These are *respiratory* clues that should prompt you to respond with a respiratory intervention. You might say that you will reposition your patient for adequate oxygenation, apply oxygen, and call the provider.

If the patient has crushing chest pain or clutches his hand to his chest, you are being provided *cardiac* clues that should prompt you to obtain a stat ECG, assess for quality and duration of pain, place on a cardiac monitor, call RRT, prepare to initiate basic life support if needed, and call the provider. If the patient arrested, you say, "Call for help and initiate basic life support."

It's a bonus (meaning good if you do this but not held against you if you don't) if you demonstrate critical thinking when answering situational interview questions. You do this by anticipating the next steps and which labs or tests the doctor will order. For example:

- If they say the patient has crushing chest pain, you might say, "Anticipate transfer to cath lab or ICU."
- If they say the patient has severe difficulty breathing, you could say, "Provide respiratory support, call a respiratory therapist, and direct someone to get the crash cart for possible intubation.'

Remember, you do not have to mention all possible interventions, and there are no hard and fast or right and wrong answers.

However, it *is highly* important to say that you will seek help from a charge nurse or RRT. That shows that you are safe, and essentially that is what they are looking for in a new grad. Nurse managers screen for nurses who do not know that they need help because it puts patients at risk.

Here are the correct responses. The best candidates included all of the following (notes taken from actual interviews):

- "I will call for help (call RRT or charge nurse)"—*shows understanding of role and safety.*
- "I will stay at the bedside"—*demonstrates safety.*

- "I will assess the patient (take vital signs, finger stick, and so on)"—*applies the nursing process and doesn't panic.*
- "I will consider the appropriate interventions (raise the head of the bed, apply oxygen)"—*shows critical thinking.*
- "I will call the provider"—*good.*
- "I will anticipate what the provider might order (cardiac enzymes, ECG, CXR, and so on)"—*better.*

To summarize, the purpose of situational interview questions is to determine if you are a safe clinician. You are not expected to be an expert and it is understood you are inexperienced.

What is important is having a teachable spirit and knowing your limits.

16

Closing the Interview and Beyond

It's no use going back to yesterday, because I was a different person then.

—Lewis Carroll, Alice in Wonderland

At the end of an interview, be prepared with your own questions. Not having any questions may lead the interviewer to assume you are not prepared, not savvy, or not interested. Asking smart, insightful questions that make you stand out from others can land you the job. Asking questions changes the dynamic and can make you appear to be weighing your options in a good way (even if it's the only interview you have lined up).

WHAT QUESTIONS DO YOU HAVE FOR US?

Be ready with at least four questions designed to show that you know about the organization, and reiterate your desire to succeed in the role. Have four because you should ask two questions, and two may have been answered during the course of the interview.

- "What steps need to be taken before an offer can be made?"
- "What are the most important characteristics of a successful nurse here at Happy Hospital?" (If asked at the beginning of an interview, you gain insight into what they're looking for, which can help guide your later responses.)
- "What are the next steps in the interview process?"
- "I know that one of the mission values is transparency. How is that manifested for employees?"
- "What is unique about the culture here?"
- "Can you describe the leadership styles here?"
- "Can you tell me about the team I'd be working with on the nursing unit?"

BONUS QUESTION

- "Can you tell me what is rewarding for you about working here?"

What makes this a bonus question? This is an especially good question as it sets you apart. Very few other competing candidates will show this level of interviewing sophistication. Second, people love to talk about themselves, and you will generate some animated responses. The mood will change to positivity and surprise in a good way. Later, you and your name will be associated with the good feelings. You will have made yourself memorable.

THINGS NEVER TO ASK

- Never ask about salary until a job offer has been extended.
- Do not ask, "Is this for day shift or night shift?" or "Will I have to work on weekends?" when you are a new grad. It may convey entitlement.
- Never mention future vacation plans or hint that you may need time off.

HOW TO STAND OUT

After the interview and within twenty-four hours, send a brief thank-you note via e-mail. Here's an example:

Hi, Beth,
   It's Marc. I had my interview with you guys on Wednesday. I came in shortly after

the lunch break. I just wanted to say thank you again for taking the time to meet with me. Everybody was so friendly and gracious. It was a pleasure meeting with you, and I hope to possibly work with you in the future. Again, thank you for the interview.

Happy recruiting!
Marc Johnson

First of all, it is short—less than one hundred words. Thank-you notes should be brief.

Next, he wrote it with me (the reader) in mind: "It's Marc. I had my interview with you guys on Wednesday." He doesn't assume I'll remember him, so he adds "the one who came in after lunch."

Then he compliments us in a genuine manner. We all like to think we're "friendly and gracious." I certainly do.

He gave a call to action: "I hope to possibly work with you in the future." This way, Marc positively reaffirms his desire to gain the position.

Finally, he signs off with "Happy recruiting!" which is creative and a touch of fun. He didn't use "thank you" again as that would have been an overuse.

Marc hit the mark. It was genuine, and the overall tone was light and sincere.

MAKE YOURSELF STAND OUT

What Marc creatively did made him stand out from *every other candidate* we interviewed that week. In this competitive market, you need to make a singular impression. How did he do it? By using simple manners and a thank-you note after his job interview.

There are four ways in which Marc stood out:

- Manners: Good manners such as sending a thank-you note never go out of style but are so rarely used that they make you stand out.
- Initiative: I did not give Marc my card or even my last name, but he managed to find every interviewer's name and e-mail address. Well done.
- Smart: He's obviously clever to think of the idea and to compose the thank-you note.
- Brief and articulate.

On the basis of his short thank-you note, I attributed many more positive attributes to him. Here's what I was thinking: *Wow, who does that nowadays? Very impressive. He's a thoughtful guy. He can write well, too, which is a sign of intelligence. Someone had to teach him that. I bet he comes from a good family;*

he knows how to conduct himself. He'd be polite and conduct himself well on the floor.

Don't underestimate the benefit of a small gesture such as a thank-you note. It takes a short time to compose and send but will be well received.

THE WAITING GAME

If you have finished your job interview and are waiting anxiously for an offer, do not put your job search on hold. Continue checking job boards, continue applying, and keep networking. Don't put all your eggs in one basket, as my grandmother used to say.

IF YOU DON'T GET THE JOB

After an interview, if you did not get the job, call and ask how to improve your interviewing skills. You may not always get feedback, but you may get some very valuable feedback. It's in the "you have nothing to lose" category. Send a short e-mail to the hiring nurse manager and ask, "Can you give me any feedback on my interview answers to help me in future interviews? Your insight would be greatly appreciated." Nurse managers who enjoy helping others develop professionally will respond, given their time restraints.

If you do not get a response from the nurse manager, try calling the hospital-based recruiter. Even though he or she may not have participated in the interview, they will have talked to the nurse manager or could do so on your behalf.

> *If you fell down yesterday, stand up today.*
>
> —H. G. WELLS

When you are not offered the job, try to take it in stride. Every interview is a skills-building opportunity. You must persevere and keep going. There are other jobs out there, and your efforts will pay off. Always work on improving your skills, but remember that you may never know all the reasons behind hiring decisions.

Some have nothing to do with you whatsoever. In higher-level jobs, it is not unheard of to conduct interviews when a candidate has already been selected. Granted, this is not usually the case in entry-level new grad positions, but the point is to try not to take it personally because often it is not personal at all.

You also may want to consider looking outside of the acute-care setting. Many nurses find wonderful, satisfying roles in public health, subacute, rehab, and outpatient clinics, to name just a few. Broaden your scope, and keep looking. Nursing is the most versatile profession on the planet.

Cultivate patience and trust. Your ship will sail.

17

Final Words and Bonus FAQs

Thank you for reading, and I really hope this guide has been helpful to you. On my site, nursecode.com, there are more examples of sample résumés and cover letters and more tips and strategies to help you wherever you are in your career.

If you are a new grad, you are going to need plenty of positive support during your first year. Read *Becoming Nursey: From Code Blues to Code Browns, How to Care for Your Patients and Yourself*, by Kati Kleber, who heartwarmingly takes you through her first year as a rookie nurse.

I included some helpful FAQs in this final chapter as an example of questions I am asked in my "Ask Nurse Beth" column at Allnurses.com, the world's largest online nursing forum. For these and any other career questions or personal career advice, please visit me at allnurses.com and submit a personal question to "Ask Nurse Beth." Here are some examples of questions I am frequently asked.

COLD-CALLING A NURSE MANAGER

Question: Is it ever OK to walk into a nurse manager's office, résumé in hand, to apply for a nursing job (cold call)?

You may have considered it, but you're not sure if it's such a wise move—not to mention it's scary! So is it bold and brassy but OK? Or risky and regrettable?

Answer: It is bold, brassy, and risky, and can be regrettable or wildly successful.

Like most risky moves, it could pay off big time or backfire big time. Some managers will see walking in to apply for a job as circumventing the process and be irritated. They may pointedly inform you to apply through HR like everyone else and dismiss you while looking down at their desktop. That's the risk. But even managers who are irritated in the moment may inwardly admire your spunk. And when your résumé comes across their desk through the usual channels, they'll remember you.

Other managers will size you up when you walk in to apply for a job and then give you a moment. If so, be brief, respectful of their time, and thank them. Say that you are aware there is a position for which you qualify, and you wanted to drop your application off in person. This is not an interview unless the manager makes it one. But always be prepared for new grad interview questions. They may be impressed enough with your initiative and presence that they expedite your application process and hire you. That's the benefit.

My personal experience? As a hiring nurse manager, this happened to me a lot. Most commonly, an employee of mine would bring someone (a friend or relative) in unannounced, and I would have to deal with it graciously on the spot. In some cultures, this is the way it's done. Jobs are obtained more by who you know than by applying.

At times, yes, I did find it irritating that my busy day was interrupted. But if it was a high-performing employee who I valued that was bringing in a friend, I tended to pay more attention and extend myself more on his or her behalf. I absolutely did hire some great employees this way.

Walking in to apply for a job has a higher chance of being effective when you have a connection with someone in the organization, but that's not to say you can't do it on your own. If you are going to do this, aim for a Monday or Friday, when meetings are predictably fewer, and there's a greater chance the nurse manager will be in the office and not in a meeting.

At the very least, you can leave your résumé, captivating cover letter, and contact information: "Hello. I understand there's an opening for a new grad nurse. I wanted to drop off my résumé in person." Difficult times call for bold moves.

AFTER MY INTERVIEW, WHEN SHOULD I CALL BACK?
Question: When Should I Call Back?

Answer: No one wants to be annoying, and most of us would rather do nothing than risk appearing pushy, overeager, or desperate. But you want to stay on their radar, and sometimes she or he who follows up lands the job.

If you were given a timeline after an interview when you will be contacted, wait three to four days after the deadline and reach out: "Hello. I hope this finds you well. I'm just contacting you to find out if there's an update yet for the job I interviewed for on November sixth. I wanted to let you know I'm still very interested and looking forward to hearing from you." If you still do not hear back, contact them again in one to two weeks: "Just following up on the previous note. Let me know when you have a moment."

Personally, I have had great results with similar follow-up and have landed two or three jobs this way. I made it easy for them to pick me. People are busy, priorities change, and some people are forgetful or unreliable. I operate from a risk/benefit "what do I have to lose?" approach. At the very least, you will have closure and know that you did the most you could do.

Once when I was working as an educator and the most junior person on the education team, corporate office announced they needed a nurse trainer in Hawaii for two weeks. Naturally, all the nurse educators applied. I did, too, but knew I didn't have a chance for such a plum assignment, as I was new.

Day after day, I kept checking my e-mail for any update. A couple of weeks dragged by and they still hadn't picked anyone. Meanwhile, I happened to attend a luau function all dressed up with a lei, Hawaiian dress, and flowers in my hair. I sent a selfie with the caption "Pick me! I'm ready to go!"

Two weeks later, my husband and I were in Waikiki making snorkeling plans. Persistence pays off.

I'M OLDER—WHAT ABOUT AGEISM?

Question: I'm a new grad but a second career nurse and am forty-nine. I'm not getting a job, while my classmates are. Could it be my age? Is this discrimination?

Answer: It's a possibility. Older people are often mistakenly seen as irrelevant, slow, and a burden on society. Likewise, there is ageism in nursing. Jobs go to younger applicants. Older nurses are squeezed out and replaced by younger ones. If you show up to an interview with wrinkles, are you automatically disqualified? Yes, you may be.

There are laws to prevent age discrimination. The Age Discrimination in Employment Act (amended in 1986) says that it's illegal for an employer to discriminate against you if you are over forty (there is no upper cap on age). However, this is not likely to help an aging nurse even if she or he is being discriminated against.

But here are some tips to help you in the workplace and when interviewing for a job.

Stereotypes

Stereotypes of older workers exist, and they can be inaccurate and damaging.

- Older nurses are slower. They cannot keep up.
- Older workers are resistant to change. They are rigid and set in their ways.
- Older workers cannot understand technology.

What you can do to mitigate age discrimination

The law is not going to help you. Age discrimination is difficult to prove even if you are inclined to spend the time and money. What you *can* do is change yourself.

Do not internalize society's views on aging. Do not draw attention to your age.

- For experienced nurses, do not repeatedly say, "Back in my day" or "When I started nursing, we had twenty-five patients and no IV pumps."
- Do not refer to yourself as old. Daily at my work, I hear coworkers brand themselves as old, and I wince.

- Resist the temptation to talk about your aches and pains or point out to others that you can no longer read up close without glasses.
- Have a positive focus. You have valuable life experience. You have a strongly established work ethic. You are not going to get pregnant. You have learned to play well in the sandbox with others.

Stay vibrant

What age are you projecting? Pay attention to your personal appearance. What is it saying about you? Is your appearance age appropriate?

- Stay fit and healthy—this is half the game. Never give up. Sit up straight with your back not touching the chair. Cultivate a spring in your step and a light in your eye.
- Project energy and enthusiasm.
- Pay attention to the vibe you are projecting and your energy aura. Energy is attractive. Be passionate. Use words like "energy" and "motivated" in your interview.

Stay relevant/stay in touch

Stay relevant in your field. Practice is changing a mile a minute. Read journals and pursue continuing education. Be known as the nurse with the latest evidence-based information. Be a lifelong learner. Intellectual curiosity is your ally.

Stay culturally relevant. For example, occasionally listen to current popular music, read books, see movies, and be aware of beauty/fashion trends. If you have a sixteen-year-old in your life (like my niece), you have an automatic pipeline to the latest everything. Try new restaurants. Be open-minded. Stay tuned in.

Create your own value

Create a niche for yourself. What does that mean? You can be the unit expert on twelve EKGs or blood gas interpretation.

You can be comfortably confident by virtue of maturity—no limp handshakes for you. You know how to make eye contact and conduct yourself socially.

Emphasize your technology skills. Put your LinkedIn URL on your résumé as a contact. If your e-mail account is AOL, change it to firstname.lastname@gmail.com.

Don't be your own worst enemy

You cannot change others, but you can change yourself and choose how to portray yourself. Do not compare yourself to others who are younger. I was at an interview where an older woman giggled and said, "Well, you young people will have to help me on the computer." Did she think she was flattering the interviewers? It was not funny, it was not cute, and she was not hired.

How about this instead? "The other day on Twitter, I read an article from *Forbes* about self-governance in nursing. Is that something you do here?"

Age discrimination may not seem like a real thing until you've experienced it. It's easy to regard growing older as something that happens to other people (old people?) and not to you. But it's a fact of life. Best wishes.

CAN I ASK FOR MORE MONEY AS A NEW GRAD?

Question: Can I negotiate for a higher salary as a new grad?

If you're a new nursing grad with a job offer, you may be wondering if it's OK to ask for more money. Will they think you're nervy if you do? Or naïve if you don't?

Answer: Even in the best of economic times, salary negotiation can be a risky proposition for most new grads pursuing entry-level positions. From the organization's point of view, they are going to invest a large sum in you to bring you up to speed. They tend to pay all new nurses the same. Exceptions can be made, and rules can be broken.

Typically, clinical (bedside) nursing pay is highly structured. Unlike some professions, entry-level pay in nursing is not as negotiable as you may wish. Pay grids are fixed and based on years of experience. Often, new grad nurses are all offered the same amount down to the penny.

Now that you understand the context, you're better prepared to decide if it is best for you to ask for more money. Prepare your case when asking for more money. You don't want to just *ask* for a higher salary when securing a new job. You want to make a strong case for why it *makes sense* for them to give you one.

You must offer something that sets you apart in value from the other twenty-two RNs in your cohort. Generally, first-career degrees are not a basis for more pay (for example, a degree in journalism). What sets you apart may be your BSN or certificates such as ACLS and PALS, which may garner you a differential. It might be that you are weighing more than one job offer and the employer you prefer is offering less, so your risk is mitigated. If you are relocating, the relocation allowance may be negotiable. Before the interview, compose your question and practice asking it.

How to ask for more money
Carefully. Your attitude must be humble and not convey any sense of entitlement.

Employ thoughtful, strategic questions like "I have my BSN. Is this something that's worthwhile to you, and, if so, are you open to negotiating a higher starting salary?" Ask once—just once. If they respond, "We don't negotiate," then nod agreeably.

It's not just about the money. Compensation packages are about so much more than hourly salary. Make a spreadsheet and compare wages, tuition reimbursement, vacation time, benefit costs, and coverage between two or more employers. Consider nonquantifiables that you are looking for like length of orientation, reputation of the hospital, and room for advancement. These are all highly important and should be factored into your decision. Does the hospital offer a clinical ladder? If so, consider applying to the clinical-ladder program as soon as you are eligible as you will earn more money.

Summary

It's true that you will never know if there's wiggle room in pay or benefits until you ask. Nothing ventured, nothing gained. I know of one young man who asked, and they immediately upped his hourly wage by fifty cents and added to his relocation expenses. It could be that they really, really wanted this candidate. What you want to know is does it hurt your chances to ask? Probably not if you do it respectfully and only after the job offer has been extended. It's highly unlikely that a nursing manager would withdraw a job offer at the last stages simply as a result of your asking.

In a very short time, you will be more marketable, and you will have much more leverage when you seek your next job. At that time, negotiating skills will really pay off.

WHAT IF I HAVE A DUI?

Question: I finished nursing school, but the BON found out I had a DUI and did not let me sit for my NCLEX exam. I'm so worried. What should I do?

Answer: So your application to the BON for initial licensure was denied due to a DUI or other offense. You now need to write a letter of explanation regarding your offense or DUI to the BRN. This letter is extremely important and must be very well written. Through your written words, they will assess your level of remorse and personal responsibility and determine your future.

Include the following information in your letter.

Detailed description of the circumstances

State what happened factually and chronologically. Don't offer excuses or cast blame, but include underlying circumstances. It can be very helpful to describe the conditions in your life at the time that affected your decisions. Most bad choices don't come out of nowhere, and people understand that.

Your insight into your own behavior here is key. Tell them what you've learned about yourself and how your values have changed.

Thorough description of the rehabilitative changes in your lifestyle

The BON wants to see that you have taken responsibility and put systems in place to ensure that there is not a reoccurrence of the problem. List everything you've done to prevent future occurrences. This can include attending a recovery program, community work, or therapy. Include compliance with terms of probation, restitution, or parole.

You may live in a different area with positive influences now, or maybe you've joined support groups. Show that you are not the same person who committed the offense.

Show remorse

You are genuinely sorry for what you did. You now know you could have harmed yourself or someone else. You can't change the past, but you can control your future behavior. You have grown from this and regret the choices you made in the past. You are remorseful.

Consider getting letter-writing help

It's best to get help from someone to write this unless you are very confident and proficient in your writing skills. Some applicants find it helpful to retain a lawyer during the process to ensure that the licensing process goes smoothly. This can be expensive, and not all attorneys accept payments over time. Start saving for legal expenses in advance if you anticipate a problem, and be patient.

Letters of reference

Letters of reference should be on official letterhead from employers, nursing instructors, health professionals, professional counselors, parole or probation officers, or other individuals in positions of authority who are knowledgeable about your rehabilitation efforts. They must be signed and dated within the past year.

What to expect

You may face probation, a conditional license with probation terms, a fine, or a citation. If your DUI was a fairly low blood-alcohol level (BAC), you may only face a letter of reprimand or a citation and fine.

Do not ignore any mail from the BRN or attorney general's office. Make sure your current address is on file at all times. Your failure to respond to the statement of issues will result in the denial of your license application by a default process.

The BRN decides on these cases individually, and the decision may take some time. A criminal history does not mean that you cannot become a nurse, but it may mean extra work and extra expenses. Best wishes.

WHAT IF I'M OFFERED ANOTHER JOB WHILE WAITING TO HEAR BACK?

Question: What if I receive another job offer while I'm waiting to hear back after an interview?

Answer: When you receive a job offer, you do not have to give an answer immediately. You can very graciously thank them for the offer and say you need some time to think about it. Provide a time frame such as "I can have an answer within five days. Will that work for you?" Now you have bought some time for yourself.

In the meantime, contact the first employers and tell them that while they are your first choice, you have received another job offer. When do they expect to make their decision? If the first employers consider you a top candidate, they will respond by making you an offer. If they do not consider you a top candidate, they will stall or respond with a lack of interest.

New grads attempting to land their first jobs have more at stake in this situation. A solid job offer trumps a potential job offer. In the end, you must weigh the advantages and disadvantages.

Conclusion

I really hope the tips and strategies in this book help you feel more prepared and confident in your job search. That's my goal in writing this book—to help get you started in your nursing career!. It's such an exciting time for you and I wish you all the best.

Finally, I hope you love your nursing career as much as I've loved mine, with the countless opportunities to grow and to help others.

> *There is freedom waiting for you,*
> *On the breezes of the sky,*
> *And you ask "What if I fall?"*
> *Oh but my darling,*
> *What if you fly?*

— Erin Hanson

About the Author

Beth Hawkes is a nurse, past nurse manager, and writer who has helped nurses through every stage of their professional development. Her blog, Nursecode.com, provides a variety of useful tips and resources for beginning or furthering a nursing career. Hawkes also writes the "Ask Nurse Beth" column at Allnurses.com, the world's largest online nursing forum.

Hawkes works as a nursing professional-development specialist. She works with the American Nurses Association, the Association for Nursing Professional Development, and the Academy of Medical-Surgical Nurses as a column editor and content developer.

Suggested Readings

Benner, P. 1984. *From Novice to Expert*. Menlo Park, CA: Addison-Wesley.

Carlson, K. 2015. *Savvy Networking for Nurses: Getting Connected and Staying Connected in the 21st Century*. Santa Fe, NM: Nurse Keith Coaching..

Kleber, K. 2015. *Becoming Nursey: From Code Blue to Code Brown, How to Care for Your Patients and Yourself*. Nurse Eye Roll LLC. Publisher: Author.

Made in the USA
Middletown, DE
06 January 2020

82695346R00119